the Strong*Curves* Cookbook

Quarto.com

© 2024 Quarto Publishing Group USA Inc.
Text © 2024 Shelley Darlington

First Published in 2024 by Fair Winds Press, an imprint of The Quarto Group,
100 Cummings Center, Suite 265-D, Beverly, MA 01915, USA.

T (978) 282-9590 F (978) 283-2742

Fair Winds Press titles are also available at discount for retail, wholesale, promotional, and bulk purchase. For details, contact the Special Sales Manager by email at specialsales@quarto.com or by mail at The Quarto Group, Attn: Special Sales Manager, 100 Cummings Center, Suite 265- D, Beverly, MA 01915, USA.

28 27 26 25 24   1 2 3 4 5

ISBN: 978-0-7603-8525-8

Digital edition published in 2024
eISBN: 978-0-7603-8526-5

Library of Congress Control Number: 2023947410

Cover Image: Mathilde Bouby
Page Layout: Mattie Wells
Photography: Mathilde Bouby
Food Photography: Alison Bickel

Printed in China

The information in this book is for educational purposes only. It is not intended to replace the advice of a physician or medical practitioner. Please see your health-care provider before beginning any new health program.

Dedication

**I dedicate this book to the women who helped shape me:
my mother, Batia, my safta, Rachel, and my nana, Audrey.
Your memory lives on in these pages.**

the StrongCurves
Cookbook

100+ High-Protein, Low-Carb Recipes to Help You Lose Weight, Build Muscle, and Get Strong!

Shelley Darlington

founder of **Strong Curves**

FAIR WINDS

Contents

Introduction 6

Chapter 1: **Pre-Workout** 28

BREAKFAST 30
Chocolate Mint Smoothie Bowl 30
Mexican-Style Egg Frittata 32
Zesty Salmon Power Bowl. 33
Full English Breakfast Quesadilla 34
Fuel-Up Breakfast Burger 36
Vanilla Protein Pudding 37

LUNCH 38
Pork San Choi Bao. 39
Warm Steak Salad 40
Ham and Egg Cups 41
Chicken and Avocado
Lettuce Wraps. 42
Egg Salad Wrap 43
Teriyaki Salmon and Bok Choy. 44
Chicken and Sweet Corn Soup 46

DINNER. 47
Italian Meatballs 47
Creamy Tuscan Chicken. 49
Chicken Shish Taouk Skewers 50
Stuffed Cabbage Rolls 52
Tuna Casserole 53
Grilled Shrimp and Zucchini Salad 54

SNACKS 56
Salmon and Cucumber Canapés. 57
Greek Yogurt and Berries. 58
Protein Bento Box 59
Blueberry and Zucchini Muffins. 60
Chewy Fig Protein Bar 62

SIDES & SALADS. 63
Chop-Chop Salad. 63
Red Cabbage Slaw 64
Sautéed Green Beans and Mushrooms. 65
Cheesy Broccoli Poppers. 66
Stuffed Mushrooms 69

Chapter 2: **Post-Workout** 70

BREAKFAST 72
Apricot Breakfast Bake. 72
Banana Protein Pancakes 74
Cherry Chocolate Masa Bowl. 75
New York Deli Breakfast Burrito 76
Japanese-Style Egg and Rice. 79
Savory Oatmeal with a
Poached Egg 80

LUNCH 81
Sweet Potato and
Turkey Quinoa Bowl 81
Shakshuka (Eggs Poached in
Tomato Sauce) 82
Crispy Shrimp Rice Paper Rolls 85
BLT Pasta Salad 86
Tuna and Mayo Topped
Baked Potato. 87
Taco Nachos with Salsa 88

DINNER. 91
Chicken Enchiladas. 91
Red Thai Curry with Shrimp 92
Salmon Sushi Bake 94
Chili Con Carne. 95
One Pan Moroccan Potato Hash 97
Beef and Rice Stuffed Peppers. 98

SNACKS 100
Sweet Potato Avocado Boats 101
Rice Cakes 3 Ways. 102
No-Bake Protein Bar 103
Cinnamon Apple with Nut Butter 104
Pesto Deviled Eggs 105

SIDES 106
Herbed Latkes. 106
Mushroom Pearl Couscous. 108
Sweet Potato Fries. 109
Bone Broth Rice 110

DRINKS AND SMOOTHIES 111
Peanut Butter Banana Smoothie 111
Green Goddess Smoothie 112
Strawberry Oatmeal Smoothie 114
Electrolyte Replenisher 115
Chocolate Malt Collagen Shake 116

SWEET TREATS 117
Protein Brownies 117
Coconut Energy Balls 118
Honey Puffed Rice Bars 120
Protein-Packed Chocolate Pudding 121
Frozen Yogurt Bites 123

Chapter 3: Rest Days   124

BREAKFAST 126
Grain-Free Porridge 126
Avo Egg Smash 127
Salmon and Cream Cheese Sushi 128
Egg and Feta Muffins 129
Grain-Free Granola 130
Blueberry Breakfast Bake 131

LUNCH 132
Shrimp-Stuffed Avocado 132
Mushroom and Bacon Soup 135
Salmon and Cream Cheese Crepes . . 136
Zucchini Fritters with Fried Eggs 137
Mini Salmon Broccoli Quiche 138
Cheesy Chicken Patties 139
Baked Spinach and Feta Tortilla 140

DINNER 141
Pork Egg Roll in a Bowl 141
Veggie Buddha Bowl 142
Butter Chicken with Cauliflower Rice . . 145
Turkey Stuffed Peppers 146
Sweet and Sour Beef 147
Zucchini and Prosciutto
"No Pasta" Lasagna 148
Pesto and Mozzarella
Stuffed Chicken 149

SNACKS 150
Cauliflower Falafel and
Tahini Dip 151
Cheesy Bacon Fat Bomb 152
Cottage Cheese and Avocado Bowl . . . 153
Spaghetti Squash Pizza Nests 154

SWEET TREATS 156
Nut Butter Buckeyes 156
Crepes with Berries and Cream 158
ANZAC Biscuits 159
Baklava Bites 160
Peanut Butter Banana Muffins 162

DRINKS 163
Sugar-Free Hot Chocolate 163
Sweet 'n Salty Fat Tea Latte 165
Healing Bone Broth 166
Adrenal Support Cocktail 167
Berry Collagen Shake 168

Notes 169
Acknowledgments 170
About the Author 171
Index 172

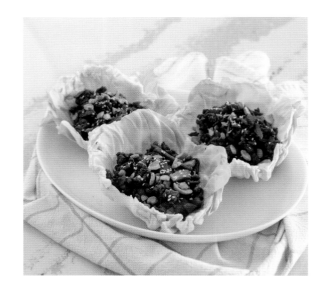

Introduction

Welcome to **The Strong Curves Cookbook**, the ultimate guide to nourishing your body with healthy, whole food recipes that support muscle building and fat loss. I'm Shelley, and I'm the founder of Strong Curves, a fitness brand that empowers women to embrace their strength, confidence, and vitality.

As a fitness expert and qualified nutritionist with over a decade of experience, I've helped countless women transform their bodies and their lives through weightlifting and proper nutrition. During that time, one thing I've consistently noticed is that many women struggle with finding healthy and delicious recipes that support their fitness goals.

As women, we face unique challenges when it comes to our health and fitness. Our bodies are different from men's, and we need specific nutrients to support our hormonal balance and overall health. That's why this cookbook is designed with YOU in mind, providing recipes that are tailored to a woman's specific needs. The recipes in this cookbook are animal-based and packed with protein, healthy fats, and complex carbohydrates to support muscle growth and fat loss through a balanced way of eating. But more importantly, they're designed to be simple and delicious, so you can enjoy them even if you're not a gourmet chef.

The Strong Curves Cookbook is divided into three chapters, each focusing on a different aspect of your fitness journey. Chapter 1 is all about pre-workout recipes, which will give you the energy and nutrients you need to power through your workouts. Chapter 2 focuses on post-workout recipes, which will help you recover and rebuild your muscles after your training. And Chapter 3 is dedicated to rest day recipes, which will help you nourish your body on your days off.

In each chapter, you'll find a variety of recipes that are easy to make, delicious, and packed with nutrients. From protein-packed smoothies and breakfast bowls to savory salads, hearty soups, and comforting stews, there's something for everyone, no matter the meal or time of day.

But the benefits of this cookbook go far beyond just tasty recipes. By following the Strong Curves approach to nutrition, you'll be giving your body the fuel it needs to build muscle, burn fat, and feel amazing. You'll have more energy, better focus, and greater endurance in the gym, and you'll see faster results from your workouts.

But perhaps most importantly, you'll develop a healthier relationship with food. You'll learn to see food not as something to be feared or avoided, but as something to be enjoyed and appreciated. You'll discover that eating healthy doesn't have to mean sacrificing taste or satisfaction, and you'll feel empowered to take control of your health and your fitness journey.

Whether you're a seasoned fitness enthusiast or just starting out on your fitness journey, The Strong Curves Cookbook is the ultimate guide to healthy, whole food recipes that support muscle building and fat loss. I hope you enjoy these recipes as much as I did creating them.

My Story

When I was a teenager, I felt anything but strong, confident, or healthy. Painfully skinny and insecure, I hated anything athletic so much that I would hide in the bathroom at school to avoid it.

In those days, I desperately wanted to feel womanly, to be like the strong and confident heroines in the movies. If you had told me then that in a couple of decades, I would have a thriving fitness YouTube channel and the privilege of sharing my fitness and nutritional expertise with hundreds of thousands of women all over the world, I would have laughed hard. Me, a fitness expert? No chance.

Yet, here I am!

Getting here was not easy. In my early twenties, I struggled with health issues stemming from a lifetime of junk food and TV dinners. I developed digestive issues, hormonal imbalances, heavy and painful periods, skin breakouts, mood swings, and low energy. My lowest point came after I had emergency surgery for a burst appendix, which led to a bad reaction and a six-week hospital stay that caused me to lose over twenty pounds from my already thin frame, leaving me dangerously underweight.

It wasn't until I made the huge (some might say crazy!) decision to move halfway across the world to start a new life in Australia that everything changed. There, I met my partner, Adam. He had been going to gyms since his early teens and excelled at sports in school—the complete opposite of me. He was a skilled strength coach who worked with elite-level athletes and believed in me in a way that no one ever had, least of all me. He was the first person to encourage me to start looking after my physical body. I had known for years that I needed to make a change, and finally, with his support, I started to do it.

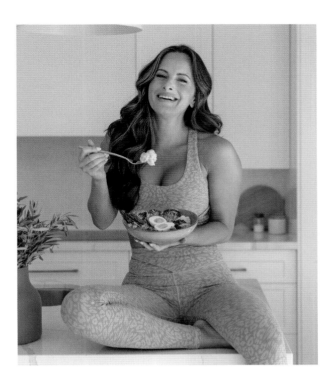

Back then, there were no fitness influencers, so I started copying Adam's eating habits, which were obviously designed to support a male body pursuing heavy body-building goals. Instead of red wine and McDonald's, I opted for steak and green beans. In a bid to become more active, I started practicing yoga. The gym terrified me—but also intrigued me. Eventually, I mustered up the courage to ask Adam if he would help me start lifting weights.

He was hesitant at first. He'd witnessed firsthand just how dysfunctional the body building industry could be for women, turning them into neurotic, diet-obsessed gym addicts—a phenomenon that has now, sadly, poisoned the masses through the rise of social media. The last thing he wanted was for me to fall prey to this unhealthy lifestyle.

But eventually, he agreed and the grounded and disciplined foundation he instilled in my training in those early days is the same foundation we now practice on the Strong Curves YouTube channel, the Strong Curves app, and now, in this cookbook. I'm going to talk about it quite a bit in the next few sections, but here it is, plainly put: the simple things, done really, really well.

It took me six months of consistent gym sessions before I noticed any significant changes in body composition, but the internal transformation happened much sooner. I felt stronger, more accomplished, and more confident. To my own surprise, I loved the process and stayed consistent by focusing on my fitness goals. To support those goals, I turned my attention to my diet. I officially abandoned junk food and red wine and started focusing on clean whole foods, following a typical bodybuilder-style diet of six meals a day, high in carbohydrates. I weighed and tracked all my food, making sure to hit my recommended caloric intake every day.

And yet . . . it didn't work. Instead of getting the toned, lean muscles I was aiming for, I gained body fat, especially around my lower belly, butt, and thighs, and had cellulite for the first time in my life. Additionally, I suffered from poor digestion, bloating, lethargy after meals, and heavy menstrual cycles. I went to see countless naturopaths and dieticians, but nothing seemed to work.

Then, I found a forward-thinking doctor who recommended a low-carb, high-fat diet (LCHF) to alleviate my symptoms. He explained the cons of consuming too many carbohydrates, even if they were "healthy" whole grains, and how important saturated fat like grass-fed butter and high-quality meat was for my metabolism and hormones. At first, I thought this way of eating was crazy. But I was desperate to feel better and willing to try anything. And it worked! Half of my symptoms disappeared overnight, and after a few months, my energy was back, my skin cleared up, and I lost the cellulite. I felt like a superhuman!

I delved deeper into the low-carb lifestyle and researched mindset training, ancestral health practices, epigenetics, and holistic living. As a woman who lifted weights and wanted to feel strong and sculpted, I realized that a low-carb diet wasn't enough to reach my goals. Although it had worked wonders for my inner health, my muscle gains and performance were still slow. There was no one in the health and fitness world talking about low-carb diets at the time (my peers were all about the "eat less, move more" approach, focusing on cardio and protein shakes) or specifically about lifting weights from a woman's perspective. So, I started to experiment on myself.

I knew from my research that animal-based whole foods were key, but what I learned from this phase of experimentation was that as women, we also need to tailor our food choices to our hormones, gut health, and body composition. While carbohydrates aren't bad for you per se, we generally eat too many for our daily needs. By finding your carb tolerance, you can ensure that your hormones are stable, you can lose weight easily, and build lean muscle at the same time.

I implemented these simple nutrition principles and started to see the muscle gains and strength I had strived for in the past. Within a year, I was competing in International Fitness and Bodybuilding (IFBB) League bikini bodybuilding shows and winning the state championships. I was eating more than 1,900 calories a day and didn't step on the treadmill once in preparation for my shows. It was a big middle finger to all the naysayers who told me it couldn't be done.

When I started my YouTube channel in 2015, my goal was to create a space where women could feel empowered and confident about their bodies. I knew firsthand the struggles and misconceptions that women faced in the fitness industry, especially when it came to nutrition. So, I began sharing my at-home workouts, fitness tips, and healthy recipe videos under the Strong Curves program, hoping to break down these misconceptions and make a positive impact.

To my surprise, my channel took off! And soon enough, I was flooded with questions about nutrition and how to eat for specific fitness goals. I understood the confusion and frustration—it took me years of research, trial and error, and perseverance to finally find what worked for me. Having already worked as a qualified personal trainer and yoga teacher for over a decade and after spending thousands of hours experimenting in the kitchen to create delicious recipes to support women who lift, I finally got qualified as a nutritionist, specializing as a health and wellness coach, in early 2023.

Why do this? It's simple. I don't want other women to go through the same struggles I did. In these days of social media, it's so easy to fall victim to misinformation. The typical fitness influencer "healthy" meal plan tends to be heavily plant-centric, low in fat, carb-heavy, and lacking in most of the nutrient-dense foods that support the female needs. While none of these foods are bad in and of themselves, combined into a full day of eating, it simply doesn't support a weight training woman's needs. A calorie restrictive diet like this may lead to some weight loss, but also comes with constant hunger, never feeling satiated, always craving either sugary foods or salty carbs, poor sleep, midafternoon crashes, and low energy. Hardly "healthy," by any measure—and certainly not sustainable.

The Strong Curves approach takes the incredible benefits of a low-carb diet and tweaks it to suit the needs of a woman who lifts weights and wants to build lean muscle while still feeling energized, strong, and healthy from the inside out. No calorie counting or tracking macros are necessary. Just eat nutrient-dense whole foods, prioritize animal-based protein, enjoy healthy fats, and learn to incorporate carbs for your unique situation. The real trick here is understanding *what* types of carbs to eat, *when* to eat them, and *how* much, based on your workout regime, your fitness goals, and your current body composition. Luckily, this cookbook has got you covered, taking all the confusion out of the process so you can just make simple and delicious meals and reach your goals with ease.

This is why I created this book. It's a culmination of my personal experience and qualified knowledge that has helped thousands of women all over the world achieve success. Through this book, I aim to provide a practical and approachable pathway for women to become masters of their bodies without gimmicks or deprivation. I want women to feel empowered and confident about their choices when it comes to nutrition and fitness.

And speaking of empowerment, that's where the name "Strong Curves" came from. To me, the name represents a celebration of the feminine body and all its beautiful curves. But it also represents the strength, both physical and mental, that women can achieve when they put their health and fitness first.

I hope this book helps you find your power and that you enjoy this collection of nourishing and delicious recipes, just as much I did creating them.

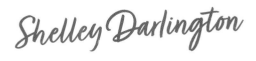

The Nutritional Science of Building Muscle

For most women practicing a weight-lifting or strength-training regimen, the goal is to gain muscle and build strength while minimizing the gaining of fat. But your time in the gym is only one part of the equation. The other part, obviously, is diet and nutrition. Unfortunately, there are countless fad diets and fitness plans out there that tout themselves as the BEST or even the ONLY way to approach this and achieve success. With this glut of information, it's hard to know what's right for your needs as a woman who lifts weights—especially if you're older, if you've crash dieted for most of your life, or if you've had children (and all the hormonal changes that come with that).

The Strong Curves approach shows you a better way to achieve your muscle building goals because as women, not only are our needs different to our male counterparts, but they are also totally individual to you. Because of this, I don't really consider the Strong Curves philosophy a diet. This isn't about imposing a set of rigid external rules on the body. Instead, we advocate a nutrient-dense, whole food, animal-based way of eating that prioritizes protein while adjusting the consumption of healthy fats and carbohydrates according to individual needs. With this nutritional philosophy as the foundation of your diet, you can do the following:

- Easily improve body composition (build muscle and lose body fat)
- Control hunger and reduce cravings (especially for sugar)
- Optimize hormones and regulate metabolism
- Improve skin and digestion
- Increase mental clarity
- Stabilize blood sugar levels for sustained energy

There are no gimmicks here—just real food tailored to the female needs. It takes a willingness to cultivate a more intimate relationship with your body and of course, to put your health first so that you become in tune with your innate bodily signals. Once you do that, calorie counting, macro tracking, and weighing your food becomes obsolete. What replaces it is true empowerment, knowing that you're nourishing your body the best way you can, while giving yourself freedom to live your life and thrive.

If you understand the basics of how your body works, how nutrition works, and what foods affect your hormones, you can in turn make better choices. And that is what we'll be focusing on in the next few sections.

A Note on Calorie Counting

Counting calories can be a useful tool for athletes who might need to shed body fat quickly. However, for the average person who just wants to look and feel their best, calorie counting is extreme and ultimately unnecessary. If you have a history of disordered or unhealthy eating or are unfamiliar with the fundamentals of nutrition, tracking your food intake can be informative and eye-opening in the short term. Starting a food diary and listing everything you eat and drink can be a helpful exercise as can tracking your calories or macros using an app, but do so only for a week or two. Using food apps as a tool can be useful, but relying on them too heavily can be counterproductive.

It's important to understand that the goal of tracking is not to become a slave to food rules or to live according to arbitrary numbers. It's simply a tool to help you understand your eating habits so you can identify any issues that need to be addressed, such as overeating or under-eating, if you're missing key nutrients, or consuming too much sugar, junk food, or alcohol. Once you have identified areas for improvement, monitor your hunger levels, satiety, cravings, energy levels, and mood to determine what changes you should make and if those changes are effective. These indicators are much better measures of success than obsessing over calorie counts.

Effortless body composition comes from optimizing your hormonal pathways, not controlling calories with calculations. Your body possesses an internal guidance system—your hunger and satiety signals—that lets you know what it needs to thrive. Certain hormones regulate these signals and those hormones are affected—negatively or positively—by the type of foods you eat.

Eat a diet full of nutrient-dense whole foods incorporating plant and animal sources and your hormonal pathways should have everything they need to function at their best. This in turn means your body can function at its best, leading to improvements in gut health, energy levels, satiety, muscle building, and fat burning capabilities. But eat a diet full of processed carbohydrates lacking in key nutrients such as animal-based protein and healthy fats and your hormonal pathways will be compromised, and you'll likely experience poor gut health, lowered immune function, and low energy. Your body's way of trying to fix this imbalance is to crave certain foods (like more carbs!) in the hopes of getting more much needed nutrients. This often results in overeating and ultimately, gaining body fat. Basically, the *quality* of your food, determines the *quantity* you eat.

Balance: The 80/20 Rule

Achieving your health and fitness goals doesn't mean you have to restrict or deprive yourself of the foods that bring you enjoyment. You should still be able to have a social life and not have to miss out on birthdays and holidays just because of your diet (this is actually a common reason many diets fail).

The 80/20 approach supports the idea of a healthy, yet balanced lifestyle. The aim is to make healthier decisions daily but also allow yourself to indulge with intention and to fully enjoy those indulgences without feeling guilty because food is fuel, but it's also about social connection and pleasure. To achieve this balance, follow the 80/20 Rule: 80% of the time eat to nourish yourself and your health and 20% of the time eat for pleasure. (These needn't be mutually exclusive. You can nourish and indulge at the same time—see my healthy sweet treats recipes in this book!)

Train, Eat, Sleep, Repeat

Before we deep dive into the core nutritional principles we'll be focusing on in this book, let's talk about how muscles actually grow. This will provide a useful framework for how and where to plug in the nutritional concepts we'll be discussing next.

The process of building muscle is threefold:

STEP 1: CHALLENGE THE MUSCLES.

You have to put your muscles under stress if you want them to grow. Cardio, high-intensity interval training (HIIT), Pilates, and yoga are great aerobic forms of exercises for heart health and general fitness, but only hypertrophy training (also known as volume training, in other words, weight-lifting) will sculpt strong curves in all the right places. Aim to lift a challenging weight and increase that weight over time with more sets and reps (progressive overload). This forces the muscle to adapt and grow.

STEP 2: FEED THE MUSCLES.

This is where this cookbook comes in! Your muscles need energy to repair and build new muscle fibers after being stressed. Animal-based protein like beef, chicken, fish, eggs, and dairy is ideal for this compared to plant-based protein due to its superior bioavailability and digestibility (more on this in a moment). Proteins break down into amino acids—the building blocks of every cell in the human body. Consuming inadequate protein will hinder muscle building, so aim for three palm-sized portions of protein per day as a good rule of thumb.

STEP 3: REST THE MUSCLES.

Muscle building and fat burning happens when your parasympathetic nervous system (PNS) is activated, triggering your body's "rest and digest" mode. This predominantly happens during sleep. For maximum gains, you need to be getting several hours of deep, delta wave-producing sleep a night (between 9 to 12 p.m. is the sweet spot). During this time, our body releases powerful fat-burning and muscle-building hormones, such as growth hormone and melatonin. If you're a light sleeper or your sleep schedule is a mess, you will neither burn fat nor build muscle to your fullest potential.

Many things can throw these important hormones out of whack and stop you entering this restorative sleep phase. The blue light from technology, which inhibits melatonin production, is a commonly recognized culprit. So is stress. Balance your hormones—and optimize your muscle gains—by getting in sync with your circadian rhythm, a.k.a. your natural sleep/wake cycle, the body's internal alarm clock that goes by the rising and setting of the sun. A few lifestyle changes that can help include: no technology two hours before bedtime, using blue light-blocking glasses after sundown, and making sure to get direct sunlight in the early hours of the day to optimize your circadian rhythm.

The Big Three (Macros)

If you only learn one thing about nutrition, let it be this: set aside the whole calories thing and instead, focus on understanding how the foods you eat affect your body and hormones. This is what will ultimately define your results. But to understand the effect of different foods on your body, you first need to have a basic understanding of the main macronutrients within those foods.

You're probably thinking, "*Wait a minute, weren't you telling me not to get hung up on nutrients or counting macros and to just focus on eating real foods?*" Yes, that's correct. However, there's no escaping the fact that we have deviated so far from our species-appropriate diet to one dominated by engineered and ultra-processed products (of which we have an overabundance of choice) that we have become disconnected from our natural eating habits and lost the ability to discern what real food even is, let alone how it affects us.

Getting a good grasp on the fundamentals will not only open your eyes to the truth about our food choices, but it will also make nutrition seem far less complicated and overwhelming. Armed with this knowledge, you can follow the Strong Curves philosophy with confidence and start to see rapid progress where you had previously only experienced plateaus.

The table at the top of the following page shows the functions of the three main macronutrients: fat, protein, and carbohydrates.

Note this table labels these nutrients as *essential* or *nonessential.* An essential nutrient is a nutrient required for normal body functioning that cannot be synthesized by the body. In other words, your body can't make its own, so you must get it from the food you eat. Carbohydrates are not considered an essential nutrient because

FAT	PROTEIN	CARBOHYDRATE
Essential nutrient	Essential nutrient	Nonessential nutrient
Breaks down into fatty acids (producing ketones)	Breaks down into amino acids	Breaks down into glucose (sugar)
Used for energy, hormone production, and brain and nervous system function	Used for energy, cell building and repair, and enzyme and antibody production	Used for energy ONLY

your body can convert non-carbohydrate sources (like the proteins and fats you eat), into glucose, a.k.a. sugar, through a process called *gluconeogenesis*. This happens mainly in the liver, but also in the kidneys and other tissues. This newly converted glucose can then be used by your body for energy or stored for later use as glycogen in the liver and muscles.

However, carbs are still an important source of energy for your body and provide other important nutrients, such as fiber and vitamins. So while they're not essential in the sense that your body can make glucose without them, they're still an important part of a healthy diet, especially for strength training women. This is why Strong Curves nutrition prioritizes animal-based protein and healthy fats first, but still includes carbohydrates (with appropriate caveats) as part of its philosophy.

Protein 101

Why is protein so important? Proteins aren't called the "building blocks of life" for nothing. It's an essential nutrient, meaning the body cannot produce it itself, so you must get it from your diet. When you eat a protein-rich food such as steak, the body breaks it down into smaller molecules called amino acids. These compounds are crucial for building and repairing every cell in your body, as well as many other vital bodily functions.

Collectively known as a *complete protein*, there are twenty different types of amino acids, and you need to make sure that you get all of them from your food in order to stay healthy. If you don't eat enough of these vital nutrients, you simply cannot function properly (let alone build muscle). This is why protein is king and why you'll see that most of the recipes in this book are so protein-centric.

DIFFERENT TYPES OF PROTEIN

Strong Curves nutrition is based on an ancestral way of eating that prioritizes the importance of an animal-based diet for optimal health and body composition. We have evolved as a species over millions of years by eating animal foods, and in my opinion, they're still the best way of meeting your protein needs. Protein is the most satiating macronutrient of the three and eating adequate amounts in your diet can help eliminate cravings and hunger.

Complete proteins are most bioavailable when they come from animal sources. Bioavailability refers to how much of a substance is absorbed by the body after it has been consumed. In the case of protein, the body absorbs and assimilates 100 percent of the amino acids found in foods such as meat, fish, eggs, and dairy. These are considered to be complete sources of protein because they contain all of the essential amino acids that your body needs to function effectively.

By comparison, sources of plant protein, such as beans, lentils, and nuts are incomplete, as they're missing some of the essential amino acids that your body needs such as isoleucine, lysine, methionine, threonine, and tryptophan.

Animal-based protein-rich foods also have an abundance of bioavailable:

- Vitamin B12: essential for making DNA, RNA, and red blood cells
- Vitamin D3: actually a hormone, only obtained from direct sunlight and meat (plant form D2 is poorly converted to D3)
- Vitamin K2: essential for bone and heart health
- EPA and DHA: brain health and nervous system function
- Cholesterol: hormones, brain, and nervous system health

HOW MUCH PROTEIN DO YOU NEED?

The leading science shows that the current recommended dietary allowance (RDA) for protein intake (0.8 grams per kilogram of bodyweight) is not enough for most people, especially for women who lift weights and whose goal is to build lean muscle mass. Between 1.2 to 2.0 grams per kilogram of body weight per day is ideal (and particularly from animal-based sources) to build muscle and stay healthy. It's also important to eat protein with every meal spread out over the entire day, rather than in one big meal. Based on three balanced meals a day, this would be 30 grams or 1 ounce of protein (or roughly a palm-sized portion of meat or fish) per meal.

However, some people do need larger amounts of protein:

- People over forty years of age with declining sex hormones, especially women who may be approaching or have been through menopause. This decline in hormones can make it harder to build muscle. Making sure to get at least 45 grams (1.6 ounces) of protein per meal sitting (or between 1.2 to 1.5 grams per kilogram of body weight) from animal-based sources is a good rule of thumb.

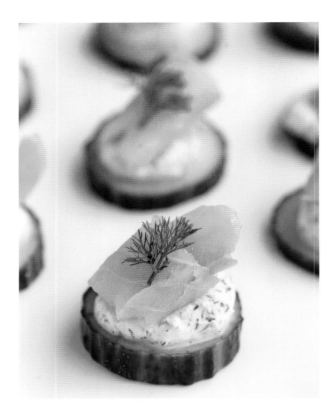

This is why weight training is even more important at this age too.

- Vegetarians and vegans who don't consume any or enough animal protein.
- Bodybuilders who are taking anabolic steroids and other performance enhancing drugs (PEDs). The use of steroids, although rampant in the fitness industry, never leads to true health. In fact, there are many dangers in using PEDs to achieve results, and for women, it is particularly dangerous as these drugs can affect your sex hormones and metabolism, causing irreversible damage and in some cases, infertility. Here at Strong Curves, we encourage the natural (and the healthiest) way of achieving results through whole foods, weight training, and stress management.

- People who have specific medical conditions and nutritional requirements.

If you don't fall under one of these conditions, as long as you eat a nutrient-dense, whole food, high-quality animal-based diet that includes meat, fish, eggs, or dairy, you can easily acquire all the essential vitamins and minerals needed to thrive without depending on expensive supplementation or worrying about hitting your recommended daily amounts. Luckily for you, this book has you covered on that front. All of our recipes for breakfast, lunch, dinner, and even our smoothies and sweet treats, are high in protein, to help you hit your recommended daily requirements whether it's a rest day or leg day at the gym!

Protein: The Bottom Line

- It's an essential nutrient for building muscle and general body functioning.
- It keeps you satiated and energized.
- Ditch the low-quality processed kind.
- Choose pasture-raised or wild-caught when possible.
- Choose whole food sources over processed supplements.
- Animal-based sources are more bioavailable and easily assimilated than plant-based sources.
- Eat a generous palm-sized portion with each meal.
- Elderly people, vegans, vegetarians, and those with specific health issues need more.

Carbohydrates 101

Carbohydrates have been demonized in recent diet culture, with many people believing that they're the cause of weight gain and other health issues. However, this is a myth that we at Strong Curves are determined to dispel. While it's true that carb consumption can impact blood sugar levels and metabolism, it's important to understand how carbs work and to consume them in moderation to support your overall health and muscle-building goals. This next section will detail the basics of carbs and how they affect your body so you can understand how to better tailor your carb intake to your needs.

HOW DO CARBS WORK?

Eating almost any food, regardless of carb content, will spike your blood sugar levels to some degree. It's a perfectly normal function of the digestive system. The issue is when you have too high a spike, too often, and it starts to negatively impact your metabolism—which is why it's best to keep your carb consumption in check, especially for women who typically have lower muscle mass and higher body fat levels.

When you eat carb-rich foods, your body breaks down those carbs into sugar, or glucose, elevating the amount of sugar in your bloodstream. That sugar has to go somewhere, either to be used for energy at that time or to be stored away for later use. To manage this, your pancreas excretes insulin (the fat-storing hormone) to help shuttle each sugar molecule out of your blood and into the cells of your muscles. The more sugar there is in your blood, the more insulin is pumped out to match it. If you eat a lot of carbs and there's a lot of sugar to deal with (more than your body needs or can store in your muscles), the excess gets stored in the liver as glycogen or converted into fatty acids to be stored as fat deposits in the body.

However, excess body fat isn't the only detrimental thing that happens when you eat too many carbs. A healthy individual will normally have just under 5 grams of sugar in the bloodstream at any one time. That's less than a teaspoon of sugar. To put things into perspective, that would be the equivalent of eating just one fruit-flavored yogurt. The American Diabetes Association recognizes that anything over the amount of one teaspoon of sugar in the bloodstream is considered pre-diabetic.

Shockingly, there's nearly eight teaspoons of sugar in a single can of soda. The average American consumes the equivalent of seventeen teaspoons of added sugar a day—that's not even counting the total amount of naturally occurring sugars from a carbohydrate-rich diet. It's easy to see how quickly you can overconsume sugar (and empty calories devoid of nutrients) on a daily basis.

Eventually, these high amounts of sugar constantly and chronically spiking your blood sugar will negatively impact your insulin function, to the point where it simply stops doing its job effectively. If you already have low muscle mass, higher body fat, and poor fitness levels, continuing to eat a high carb diet, regardless of your calorie intake, will likely result in poor health, stalled weight loss, and little-to-no results.

FUEL IN THE TANK

Here's a simple analogy to help you understand it in easier terms:

Think of the carbs you eat as pure energy. Digested carbs get broken down into sugars (glucose). That glucose is fuel and your muscles are a tank. Any glucose that gets shuttled into your muscles gets converted to glycogen (basically a stored sugar molecule that's ready to be used for energy). The storage of glycogen in muscles is important for athletic performance, as

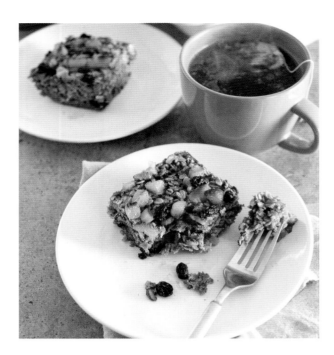

it provides a quick source of energy for the muscles to use during exercise.

Every time you train intensely with weights, you burn the fuel (glycogen) in your tank (muscles) and the tank gets depleted. So let's make a logical assumption that the more muscle you have, the bigger the capacity you have to keep fuel in the tank. That's why a 100-kilogram (220-pound) male bodybuilder can tolerate higher amounts of carbs in his diet, compared to a 60-kilogram (132-pound) woman who has higher levels of body fat and far less muscle.

Basically, the bigger the tank, the more fuel you can handle, that is, the more muscle mass you have, the more carbs you can tolerate. This is one of the key differences in men's and women's nutrition when it comes to building muscle and why it's so important for women not to copy their male counterpart's meal plans (like I was doing in the early days). Plainly speaking, you do not need as many carbs as he does.

Now, if you're continually topping up the tank with more fuel than you need, what happens?

The tank will spill over. That overflow of fuel needs to go somewhere, so where does it end up? The reserves, where it's stored as fat. So if you have a large amount of body fat to lose (lots of fuel in reserve), it would be best to limit your carbs and allow your body to use your own fat stores as fuel instead. In these cases, by eating fewer carbs, you can switch from being a sluggish sugar-burner to a highly revved up fat-burning machine.

If you don't have that much fuel in reserve, meaning you have lower body fat levels and/or more muscle, you'll be able to tolerate carbs better. In this case, the best time to refill the tank (consume carbs) is after you've depleted it from working out. The rate at which the tank gets depleted depends on the intensity and effectiveness of your workouts.

As a general rule:

- The harder you work out, the more carbs you should take in to refill the tank (think larger muscle groups worked during a lower body workout with squats and deadlifts).
- If you train smaller muscles groups, you won't need as many carbs (think upper body workouts like shoulders or abs with lighter weights).
- If it's rest day, yoga, or cardio only, your carbohydrate requirements will be even lower because your tank doesn't get depleted much at all.
- But if you have high body fat levels (lots of fuel in reserve), you don't need to refuel with carbs at all because your body can use its own stored energy more effectively.

Here's the gist of it. How many carbs you should eat is dictated by a) how much muscle vs. body fat you have and b) how often and how hard you train. Rather than seeing this way of eating as carb restriction, understand that it's about carb tolerance and timing. It's the type of carbohydrates you eat and, more importantly, when you eat them that is the key.

HOW MANY CARBS SHOULD I EAT IN A DAY?

There is no one-size-fits-all number. Your optimal carbohydrate intake depends on a combination of things such as the following:

- Age
- Gender
- Activity levels
- Body composition
- Metabolism and gut health
- Fitness goals
- Food culture

For women with low muscle mass and high body fat, Strong Curves nutrition suggests a daily carb intake that is less than the recommended Standard American Diet. That is based on my research, my experience in the fields of nutrition and fitness, and the works of prominent doctors in the field of low-carb nutrition (see Notes section at the back of this book for further details). To build muscle and lose body fat, your carb intake should depend on your current body composition, fitness level, and metabolic health. The bottom line is, the more muscle and less body fat you have, the more carbohydrates you'll be able to tolerate. In this case, there is no need to completely cut out carbs, but rather find your own carb tolerance and time your carb-heavier meals around your workouts accordingly.

NOTES FOR STRICT LOW-CARB OR NO-CARB READERS

If you're very overweight and have metabolic syndrome, insulin resistance, and/or have type II diabetes, you're probably very sensitive to eating carbohydrates. Most of the recipes in chapter 3 are lower in carbohydrates and/or keto-friendly for those who want to restrict carbohydrates for health and weight loss purposes. Where appropriate, low-carb substitutes may be offered within the higher carb recipes in chapters 1 and 2 and will be detailed in the recipe notes.

Eating fewer carbs than you might be used to can come with some unpleasant, but temporary, side effects. It's important to note that any drastic changes to your diet can have unwanted side effects—not just going lower on your carb intake! Which is why, at Strong Curves, we recommend slow and sustainable changes over long periods of time, in order to minimize any side effects. With this in mind, it's important to note that if you follow a strict low-carb or ketogenic diet, you'll lose electrolytes, including sodium, potassium, and magnesium, through urine. This excess secretion happens when your body switches over to burning fat, rather than sugar (a.k.a. the state of ketosis). An electrolyte imbalance can cause muscle cramps, fatigue, and headaches. Consuming adequate electrolytes through food or supplements is important to maintain optimal health when following a low-carbohydrate diet.

HIGH GI VS. LOW GI CARBS

Some carbohydrates have a higher Glycemic Index than others. The Glycemic Index (GI) is a rating system for carbohydrates: the higher the GI value, the higher the blood sugar spike you get from eating them. One of the principles of Strong Curves nutrition is to balance blood sugar levels no matter your goals. So, it's important to understand which foods stabilize or spike your blood sugar when determining your own individual carb tolerance.

> The Glycemic Index (GI) is a ranking system of carbohydrates in foods according to how they affect blood glucose levels, ranging from 0 to 100. Carbohydrates with a low GI value (55 or less) are more slowly digested, absorbed, and metabolized and cause a lower and slower rise in blood glucose and usually, insulin levels.
>
> —Glycemic Index Foundation

SUGAR	STARCH	FIBER
High GI fruit and fruit juices	White potato, sweet potato, and yam	Low GI fruit (strawberries, blueberries, raspberries, and blackberries)
Jam, chutney, and relish	Corn and peas	Coconut
Natural sweeteners (100% pure maple syrup, raw honey, agave, and coconut sugar)	Lentils and legumes	Lemons and limes
Store-bought sauces, dressings, and condiments	Squash and pumpkin	Tomato
Ice cream and cow's milk derived products	Beetroot, carrot, celeriac, parsnip, taro, and turnip	Cucumber
Candy, chocolate, and all confections	All other starchy vegetables	Avocado
Soda, energy drinks, beer, and cider	Rice, quinoa, and couscous	Bell pepper
Store-bought cereals, muesli, and granola bars	Oats, wheat, rye, and barley	Olives
Packaged and processed carbs	Pasta, bread, and other flour-based processed products	Mushrooms
		Nuts and seeds
		Raw cacao powder
		Onion, leek, and garlic
		Leafy greens and cruciferous vegetables

StrongCurves

DIFFERENT TYPES OF CARBS ACCORDING TO THE GLYCEMIC INDEX

The table on the opposite page shows the three main types of carbohydrates and which types of foods fall under the three categories. Sugars and starches rank high on the glycemic index, which is why it's best to enjoy these in moderation and ideally on the days you work out and more specifically, in your post-work-out meals as your carb requirements will be higher on those days. Fiber-rich foods score the lowest on the glycemic index, making them the ideal type of carbs to have on your rest days when your carb requirements are lower. Obviously, fiber-rich foods are incredibly healthy so they don't need to be limited to rest days only—enjoy them any day of the week!

Carbs: The Bottom Line

- Lower your carb consumption to stabilize blood sugar.
- Ditch the processed kind.
- Eliminate added sugars.
- Choose whole food versions.
- Time carbs around your workouts.
- Keep carbs low if very overweight.
- Increase electrolytes, especially when exercising.

Dietary Fats 101

Dietary fat is another nutrient that has come in for an unfair amount of criticism in Western food culture over the past few decades, despite being an essential nutrient for a healthy and balanced diet.

The truth is all fats are not created equal, and just like carbohydrates, it's important to distinguish between the different types.

There are four types of dietary fats (not counting trans fats—the "junk food" one), and each fat-rich food contains a combination of these types. For example, coconut oil has the highest concentration of saturated fat, but also contains small amounts of monounsaturated and polyunsaturated fats.

WHY DO WE NEED FATS?

When you consume high-fat foods such as avocado or butter, they're broken down into fatty acids in the body. Fats can be used for energy, but they play a far more crucial role within the body than just fuel. Like proteins, they're also classed as an essential nutrient, so if you don't eat enough, you'll run into problems.

Fats are crucial for the following:

- Nutrient absorption: particularly fat-soluble vitamins from plant foods. Fats help your body to assimilate and use the nutrients from your food more effectively.
- Immune functioning: strengthening your body's defense system.
- Cell signaling: allowing your body's internal communication system to run smoothly.
- Hormone production: essential to optimal well-being, weight management, and muscle building, especially for women.
- Insulation and energy storage: healthy levels of body fat is an important survival mechanism.

Not getting enough dietary fats can lead to hormone disruption, loss of your menstrual cycle, infertility, and a host of other serious health complications, which is why women shouldn't fear eating fat-rich foods. It just goes to show that, once again, women's

ENJOY	ENJOY	ENJOY	LIMIT OR AVOID	AVOID
Saturated (the "unjustly demonized" one)	Monounsaturated (the "avocado" one)	Polyunsaturated (the "Omega-3" one)	Polyunsaturated (the "Omega-6" one)	Trans (the "junk food" one)
Butter and ghee	Olives and olive oil	Fatty fish and seafood	Vegetable and seed oils	Processed products
Cream	Avocado and avocado oil	Pasture-raised meats		Baked goods
Coconut cream	Nuts	Dairy		Junk food and takeout
Coconut oil	Lard and tallow	Pasture-raised eggs		Margarine and processed spreads
Cheese		Chia, flax, and hemp seeds		
Lard and tallow		Walnuts		

needs are different than men's, who more often thrive eating the typical "high-carb, low-fat" diet touted by the mainstream fitness industry as optimal for all.

HOW MUCH FAT SHOULD I EAT IN A DAY?

According to the 2020–2025 Dietary Guidelines for Americans, the recommended daily intake for adults is 20 to 35 percent of total calories from fat. For women who lift weights, I'd actually recommend a little more than this, knowing how important dietary fats are to female needs. The great thing about eating foods high in healthy fats is that they're satisfying and give you sustained energy throughout the day—a huge advantage when actively trying to maintain a healthy weight without needing to count calories or track macros.

We know that protein requirements generally stay pretty much the same from meal to meal, and carbs fluctuate according to your activity levels. Dietary fat can simply fill in the gaps. Eat it moderately until you feel satiated. There's no need to gorge yourself on it, but there's equally no need to scrupulously limit yourself either. The beauty of high-fat foods is that they naturally regulate your appetite, so overeating doesn't tend to be an issue, especially if you're eating enough protein.

Basically, feel free to enjoy a dollop of full-fat cream in your coffee, scoop a heap of guac onto your plate, and don't be scared to melt a spoonful of butter on your steamed vegetables at dinner—but avoid unhealthy trans fats found in junk food and processed foods.

A NOTE ON SEED AND VEGETABLE OILS

Oils including canola, soybean, and corn oil are high in Omega-6 fatty acids. While Omega-6 fatty acids are essential for human health and are found in many healthy whole foods such as nuts and seeds, excess consumption can lead to an imbalanced Omega-6 to Omega-3 ratio, which has been linked to various health problems, including heart disease, cancer, and autoimmune diseases. Unfortunately, the Standard American Diet relies heavily on processed food products, which has led a majority of people to consume excess amounts of Omega 6 fats without even knowing it, while they simultaneously cut down on health-promoting Omega 3 rich foods such as red meat and eggs.

Vegetable and seed oils are also often heavily processed and refined, which can damage the fats and produce harmful compounds, such as trans fats and free radicals, that can contribute to inflammation and oxidative stress in the body. Some advocates argue that these processing methods can strip the oils of essential nutrients, such as vitamins and minerals, which are important for overall health.

While some studies support the negative impact of vegetable and seed oils on health, the scientific community is divided on this issue. Here at Strong Curves, we advocate animal-based whole food sources of dietary fats, including saturated fats from animal fats, as well as plant oils like coconut oil and olive oil over seed and vegetable oils, as they're less processed and closer to our natural species-appropriate diet.

Structuring Workouts and Meals for Best Results

Now that you have a deeper understanding of the Strong Curves principles and how the big three macronutrients affect your hormones and overall health, we can take that theory and turn it into practical steps, so you can start eating and training for your goals.

The book is already laid out in easy-to-follow chapters (Pre-workout, Post-workout, and Rest Day recipes), which form the basis of a well-balanced workout and diet plan. But here's a breakdown of how it works.

Note: Almost all your meals on training days, including snacks, drinks, and sweet treats, can be from chapter 1. The one exception, obviously, is your higher-carb post-workout meal, when you need to refuel your muscles after training.

Dietary Fats: The Bottom Line

- Essential for brain, hormones, and immune function.
- Keeps you satiated and energized.
- Don't be scared of saturated fat.
- Avoid trans fats (processed food, baked goods, and margarine spreads).
- Balance Omega-3 to Omega-6 fats.
- Avoid processed seed and vegetable oils.

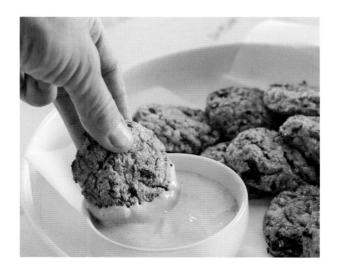

On Training Days:

BEFORE YOUR WORKOUT, CHOOSE A PRE-WORKOUT MEAL FROM CHAPTER 1.

If you're a super-early morning gym go-er, you may not feel like eating anything before your workout. That's totally okay! Just do your session and then choose a carb-rich post-workout meal from chapter 2. Or if you do need something light, pick one of our easy breakfasts or something from the snack section. Even a simple protein powder supplement shake will do.

But if you train later in the day, it's best to fuel yourself for the session ahead. The recipes in chapter 1 are designed to give you energy through healthy doses of protein and fiber, but include smaller servings of fats so you don't feel sluggish during your session. Try the Teriyaki Salmon and Bok Choy on page 44 or the Chicken Shish Taouk Skewers on page 50.

> **Pre-Workout** = High Protein, High Fiber, Moderate Carbs + Fats
> *(for all meals on training days, except post-workout)*

AFTER YOUR WORKOUT, CHOOSE A POST-WORKOUT MEAL FROM CHAPTER 2.

If you're depleting your glycogen stores, your carb requirements will naturally be higher for the day. Enjoy a moderate amount of all types of carbohydrates, including grains and starchy vegetables, but ideally, have them after intense workouts only. Remember, it's the intensity of your session that matters!

If your workout was light, maybe working small muscle groups like shoulders, arms, or core, you won't need a huge amount of carbs. A smaller serving of a starchy vegetable like sweet potato, yams, potatoes, and corn, or legumes like beans or chickpeas, is ideal. But if your day included a more intense session of heavier exercises like squats or deadlifts, then you'll tolerate more carbs, so feel free to enjoy a bigger portion of rice, oats, or pasta.

Timing carb-heavier meals after intense workouts will ensure the body uses its energy more efficiently by giving the muscles the fuel they need, exactly when they most need it. This is the most effective way to build lean muscle while minimizing fat gain.

Whether you're an early riser or late night gym junkie, we've got an array of post-workout meals to choose from like, the New York Deli Breakfast Burrito on page 76 or the Crispy Shrimp Rice Paper Rolls on page 85. Combine any of these with any of the delicious high-carb sides (page 106) for a complete, satisfying refuel meal.

> **Post-Workout** = High Protein, Higher Carbs, Lower Fats
> *(timed around your workout only, ideally after a more intense gym session)*

On Rest Days:

CHOOSE ALL YOUR REST DAY MEALS FROM CHAPTER 3.

Seeing as your activity levels are low, your carb requirements will also be lower. Even if you like to do some sort of movement on your rest day like gentle cardio or yoga, you won't need carb-rich meals because aerobic exercise doesn't deplete glycogen stores. What your body does need during this time is nourishing fats and protein to help support your hormones and stabilize your blood sugar. Coincidently, our rest day meals are also perfect during your

DO THIS PRE-WORKOUT	DO THIS POST-WORKOUT	ON REST DAYS	AVOID THIS ALWAYS
Nutrient dense whole foods	Nutrient dense whole foods	Nutrient dense whole foods	Processed products and supplements
80/20 rule with occasional indulgences	80/20 rule with occasional indulgences	80/20 rule with occasional indulgences	Calorie counting, restriction, and macro tracking
Lean protein (red meat, chicken, turkey, and white fish)	Lean protein (red meat, chicken, turkey, and white fish)	Fatty fish, seafood, eggs, and pasture-raised meat	Processed and deli meats
High-quality dairy and healthy fats (in moderate amounts)	High-quality dairy and healthy fats (in small amounts)	High-quality dairy and healthy fats (in abundance)	Low-fat dairy products, margarine spreads, and vegetable and seed oils
Leafy greens, fibrous and starchy vegetables, and beans and legumes	Whole grains, starchy and root vegetables, and beans and legumes	Leafy greens and fibrous vegetables	Refined grains and sugars
Low GI fruit (in moderation)	High GI fruit (in moderation)	Low GI fruit (in moderation)	Multiple portions of high GI fruit and fruit juices daily
Nuts and seeds (in moderation)	Nuts and seeds (in moderation)	Nuts and seeds (in moderation)	Store-bought peanut butter high in seed oils, sugar, and additives
Water, herbal tea, and coffee	Water, herbal tea, and coffee	Water, herbal tea, and coffee	Alcohol, soda, and energy drinks
Treats made with artificial sweeteners like stevia or small amounts of natural sugar	Occasional high-quality natural sweet treats (70% chocolate, raw honey, and dried fruits)	Zero-sugar treats made with artificial sweeteners like stevia	Sugar and all store-bought confections

menstrual bleed to help combat premenstrual syndrome (PMS), when you're likely to take more time off from exercising.

While you might feel the after-effects of the previous day's workout with a larger appetite than normal, high-protein and fat-rich meals will keep you feeling satiated. Pairing meals like this with fiber-rich sides, in the form of leafy greens and fibrous veggies as well as nuts and seeds, makes for a perfectly balanced day of eating. Try the Mushroom and Bacon Soup on page 135 or the Veggie Buddha Bowl on page 142.

Rest Days = High Protein, Higher Fats, Lower Carbs
(for all meals on days you rest or stay lightly active)

Meal Planning

Meal planning around a workout routine is essential for maximizing the results of your training and maintaining a healthy, balanced diet. Fortunately, meal-planning is simple and straightforward with *The Strong Curves Cookbook* because of our three chapter structure: Pre-Workout, Post-Workout, and Rest Day.

Here are some things to consider:

TIMING OF YOUR WORKOUTS

When planning your meals, it's important to consider the timing of your workouts. If you're planning to exercise in the morning, and you do want to eat something, choose a pre-workout meal that is light and easy to

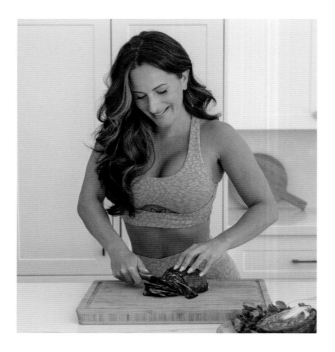

digest, such as the Chocolate Mint Smoothie Bowl or the Mexican-Style Egg Frittata, which are packed full of protein-rich ingredients such as almond milk, banana, eggs, and protein powder to fuel your workout.

Take a look at each of the three chapters with your workout regime in mind and more specifically, what time of day you'll be training. Then, simply choose whichever recipe takes your fancy from either the breakfast, lunch, or dinner sections. There's snacks, sides, sweet treats, and drinks too.

YOUR DAILY INTAKE

While it's not necessary to count calories or track your macros to get results, it's important to make sure you aren't under-eating or overeating for your needs. Everyone's daily intake and requirements will differ depending on goals, activity levels, and body composition and will vary day by day. Aside from activity levels, factors such as stress, lack of sleep, mental load, and your menstrual cycle can all affect your hunger levels and nutrient requirements.

All of this to say, it's far more important to listen to your bodily signals than to adhere to an arbitrary number of calories. Still, you should aim for a rough ballpark amount every day to ensure you're getting adequate nutrition to support your health and your fitness goals. Luckily, all the recipes in this book have been formulated with this in mind. If you follow Strong Curves recipes for your three main meals, with a choice of sides, a couple of snacks, and even a sweet treat if you fancy, you can rest assured that you'll have eaten a well-balanced and nutritious full day's caloric intake.

PLAN AHEAD

Look at the recipes and create a shopping list for the ingredients you'll need for the week. Take note of the quantities needed, so you don't end up with excess ingredients that may go to waste. It's also important to pay attention to portion sizes and divide foods up appropriately—kitchen scales are very useful for this purpose.

Next, set aside some time to prep ingredients ahead of time, such as chopping vegetables, cooking grains, and marinating meats. This can save time during the week when you're busy and may not have the luxury of preparing meals from scratch. I usually do this on Sunday afternoons after grocery shopping at the weekend farmer's market.

To make meal planning more manageable, consider batch cooking, which involves making large quantities of food at once to eat throughout the week. A slow cooker might seem like an expensive investment, but it's so worth it! This can be helpful for busy individuals who don't have a lot of time to cook during the week. Simply divide the batch-cooked meals into individual servings and store them in the fridge or freezer.

Lastly, don't forget to add some variety to your meals by trying out new recipes or experimenting with different flavor combinations. Eating healthy doesn't have to be boring, and this book offers plenty of delicious recipes to keep your taste buds satisfied while fueling your body with nutritious foods.

Adapting Your Fitness Plan for Your Monthly Cycle

Historically, the fitness industry has been largely dominated by men and rife with rigid workout regimes that favor attitudes like "go hard or go home!" or "no days off!" Because of this, women have been brainwashed into thinking that in order to get results, they too, must adopt a harsh, inflexible approach. But this couldn't be further from the truth.

Men, who live by a 24-hour daily hormonal cycle and have higher testosterone levels, do well with a regimented daily routine. Their energy levels are relatively stable day in and day out, which means they thrive on doing the same workouts for months on end. Have you ever tried to stick to a grueling gym routine, only to burn out within 6 weeks, feeling like you never really made progress despite your best efforts? Well, there's a reason for that.

Women are simply built differently. Because our bodies are on a 28-day hormonal clock, our energy levels, hormones, and bodily needs go through four distinct phases that ebb and flow every single month. Naturally, as a woman, how you move and nourish yourself should change to compliment these monthly cycles.

So, how do these four phases affect you as you move through your month, and how should you structure your workouts and adjust your nutrition to suit these shifts? Let's jump in.

The Four Phases of Your Cycle

MENSTRUAL (DAY 1–5)

This is the time during your cycle where you bleed (duration can vary between 3 to 8 days). Because the hormones estrogen and progesterone are at their lowest at this time, so are your energy levels. You'll feel tired, lethargic, and probably experience PMS symptoms like bloating, cramps, back pain, and tender breasts. Unsurprisingly, this is not the best time to lift with any intensity or try to smash personal records! Instead, take this time to prioritize self-care. These are days for bubble baths, naps, and cozy nights in with a good book. Try journalling to declutter your mind and set some intentions for the month ahead.

Recommended Exercise:

Full rest, gentle low impact cardio, yin-style yoga, or general stretching is recommended during this phase. Depending on your PMS symptoms, you may start to feel better in the latter days of your menstrual cycle. In this case, there's nothing stopping you from doing a weights session at the gym, as long as you feel up to it. Just remember, your strength levels will be lowered during this time, so don't get discouraged if you can't perform like you did in the previous weeks. Any movement is good for you, but don't push it.

Recommended Nutrition:

Try to limit carb-rich foods like pasta, bread, and potatoes according to your activity levels. Warm and nourishing foods high in protein and healthy fats will keep you satiated and help curb cravings as much as possible.

Check out the Rest Day recipes on pages 124–167 for delicious low-carb meals and snacks that will help you feel good during this time. You may feel extra hungry during this phase, especially for sweet or salty foods. Don't feel guilty for indulging more than you usually would during this time. Your body is signaling that it needs more fuel as it's working overtime on the inside.

FOLLICULAR (DAY 1–13)

This phase starts when your period begins (yes, it encompasses your menstrual phase) and lasts around 2 weeks. During this time, several follicles (fluid sacs containing an egg) are in different stages of growth. Follicle stimulating hormone (FSH) is released to prepare an egg for possible fertilization just in time for the ovulation phase. The hormones estrogen and testosterone start to rise and so does your energy levels. When estrogen peaks in the latter half of this phase (after your bleed), you'll find that your mood improves, your focus is sharper, and your libido returns. This is a great time to get sh*t done.

Recommended Exercise:

With your strength in full swing after your bleed, you can get back to lifting heavier weights and challenging yourself in the gym. This is prime muscle-building time! Focus on compound exercises like squats, deadlifts, hip thrusts, and overhead press. Aim to smash your personal records and test your strength. But a word of caution: high estrogen can make for more lax tendons and joints, so be careful if lifting heavy weights. To avoid possible injury, make sure you spend a little extra time warming up with mobility drills.

Recommended Nutrition:

As your activity levels increase, so should your food intake. However, rising hormones tend to lead to a decrease in appetite during this phase. If your goal is to build muscle, it's important to make sure you aren't under-eating, especially if you're exercising intensely. After your heavy compound lifts, your body will benefit from some more carb-rich foods, so make sure you take advantage of our Post-Workout Recipes in chapter 2.

Eating plenty of vegetables, nuts, seeds, eggs, and fish will support follicular development and help you metabolize all that extra estrogen effectively. Try the Veggie Buddha Bowl on page 142 for a lighter yet nourishing meal on a rest day during this phase.

OVULATION (DAY 14)

Ovulation is the most fertile time in the menstrual cycle, which happens around day 14 for most women. The follicle containing an egg bursts, releasing the egg into the fallopian tube. Estrogen and testosterone levels are at their highest, causing a spike in luteinizing hormone (LH). You'll likely still be riding the wave of the latter part of your follicular phase where you experience a boost in energy levels, improved mood, and an increase in sex drive. But you may also experience some abdominal bloating, breast tenderness, and cramps as you move into the next phase of your cycle.

Recommended Exercise:

If you're still feeling strong and full of energy, strength training with a little more intensity is great. Whether you push yourself with heavier weights or aim for more sets and reps, get that heart pumping! Try full body, circuit-style workouts with some walking lunges thrown in. You may find that you can push yourself harder during this phase, leading to better muscle gains and increased strength. However, if you're experiencing any discomfort or symptoms like bloating and breast tenderness, listen to your body. There's no shame in taking it a little easier too.

Recommended Nutrition:

It's important to maintain a balanced diet that includes adequate protein, complex carbohydrates, and healthy fats. You might experience an increase in appetite as your energy and activity levels increase, so it's crucial to fuel the body properly. Foods rich in iron, such as leafy greens and lean meats, like turkey, chicken, and white fish, can help combat fatigue and boost energy levels. Additionally, increasing intake of vitamin B6-rich foods like milk, cheese, tuna, sweet potato, and banana can help alleviate symptoms like bloating and breast tenderness. Try the post-workout Banana Protein Pancakes on page 74 or the Sweet Potato and Turkey Quinoa Bowl on page 81.

LUTEAL (DAY 15 TO 28)

During the luteal phase, the body prepares for pregnancy by thickening the lining of the uterus, which is facilitated by the hormone progesterone. Progesterone also helps regulate your menstrual cycle and maintain a healthy pregnancy. Both progesterone and estrogen peak with ovulation, but if pregnancy does not occur, both hormones then drop, as the body sheds the uterine lining, leading to the start of a new menstrual cycle. As you approach the latter end of your cycle, your energy and strength levels will start to drop and your core body temperature rises slightly. Don't beat yourself up if you can't perform like you had in the previous weeks. It's totally normal to experience lowered motivation during this time so be kind to yourself!

Recommended Exercise:

Working out might feel like a challenge during this phase, so it's essential to listen to your body and adjust your exercise routine accordingly. Low to moderate intensity exercise like vinyasa flows or hatha-style yoga and steady state cardio can help alleviate symptoms like bloating and cramps. You may want to avoid higher intensity workouts altogether, but if you feel up to it, try lighter weights and focus on honing your mind-muscle connection. The goal is to move your body, not to push it to the limit. Don't feel guilty for taking more rest days than usual either! Your body needs it.

Recommended Nutrition:

As you may feel more hungry during this phase, it's important to make sure you're getting enough nutrients while your body is working overtime on the inside. Eating foods rich in magnesium, like leafy greens and nuts, can help alleviate symptoms like bloating and improve mood. Adding healthy fats, such as avocados and salmon, will help regulate your hormones and nourish your body, especially on rest days from the gym. Make sure to stay hydrated and limit caffeine and alcohol intake as they can worsen your PMS symptoms. Try the Salmon and Cream Cheese Sushi on page 128 or the Baked Spinach and Feta Tortilla on page 140.

A Final Note on Your Menstrual Cycle and Your Exercise and Nutrition Plan

Not all menstrual cycles are the same or last the same number of days. The above information is only a guide. That's why it's important to really listen to your own body to work out how your unique phases feel during every month.

1

Pre-Workout

High Protein, High Fiber, Moderate Carbs + Fats

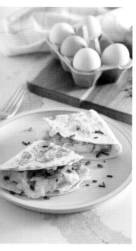

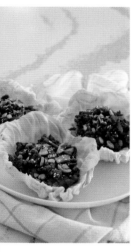

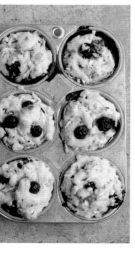

Some people prefer to train fasted on an empty stomach, especially if it's an early morning workout. But for those who need some extra energy before pumping up at the gym, these pre-workout options are satisfying, but still light—because the last thing you want is to feel sluggish and sleepy mid-session!

High protein meals with healthy fiber are lighter and easier to digest while staving off the grumbly tummy. Packed full of amino acids, these recipes provide crucial fuel to help promote muscle growth. Keeping your fats and carb-heavy foods lower before your workout is the most efficient way to deplete your glycogen stores (remember the fuel in the tank analogy!) for optimal muscle building and fat burning.

It's recommended to eat no less than 1½ hours before a gym workout to allow your body to digest your food fully; otherwise, you might feel a little nauseous and sluggish during your workout.

Chocolate Mint Smoothie Bowl

This creamy and thick smoothie bowl is a delicious start to your day. It might taste like dessert, but it's high in protein, nutrient-dense, and a satisfying way to power up for your next workout . . . and it only takes 5 minutes to make. Win-win!

Instructions:

1. In a blender, combine the avocado, frozen banana, protein powder, raw cacao powder, peppermint extract, almond milk, and ice. Blend until smooth and creamy.

2. Pour the smoothie into a bowl and sprinkle with shredded coconut. Garnish with fresh mint leaves.

3. If you prefer a thicker smoothie bowl, use less almond milk or add more ice.

Notes

Please be aware that any ingredient additions, omissions, or substitutions will affect the nutritional information.

- If you tolerate dairy, you can use full-fat cow's milk in place of nut milk.
- When choosing a protein powder, use a high-quality, clean protein powder from grass-fed cows with no additives, fillers, gums, or anti-caking agents.
- You can also add a tablespoon of chia seeds (13 g) or hemp seeds (9 g) for extra protein and fiber.
- For a sweeter taste, add a few drops of either keto-friendly stevia or a natural sweetener such as coconut sugar or raw honey.
- For a keto-friendly option, simply omit the banana and use 1 full avocado instead of half.
- Feel free to adjust the peppermint extract to your taste preference.

Difficulty: **Easy**

High Protein | Low Sugar | Gluten Free | Grain Free | Dairy Free | Keto Friendly (optional)

Prep Time | 5 minutes

Total Time | 5 minutes

Yield | 1 serving

Calories Per Serving | 406

Total Carbs | 34 g

Net Carbs | 23 g

Protein | 25 g

Fat | 20 g

Ingredients:

½ ripe avocado

½ frozen banana (see notes)

1 scoop chocolate protein powder (see notes)

1 tablespoon (5 g) raw cacao powder

¼ teaspoon pure peppermint extract

½ cup (120 ml) unsweetened almond milk or any nondairy milk of your choice

¼ cup (60 ml) ice cubes

1 tablespoon (5 g) unsweetened shredded coconut

Fresh mint leaves, for garnish

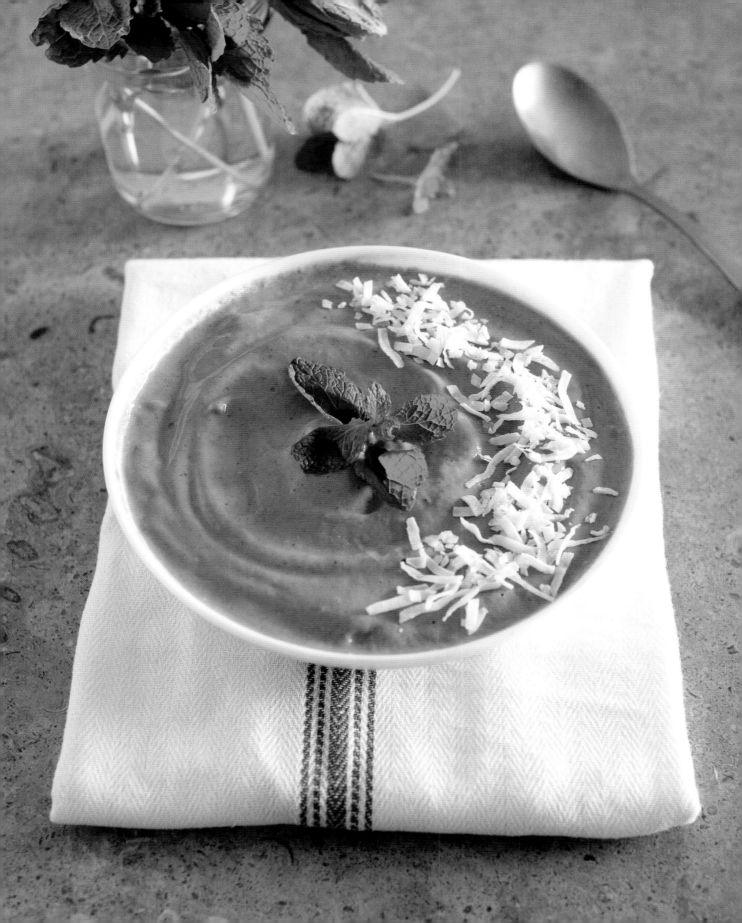

Mexican-Style Egg Frittata

This easy, flavorful frittata is the perfect high-protein breakfast to fuel you up before your next workout. Loaded with veggies and spices, it's a satisfying and healthy option that you can whip up in no time.

Instructions:

1. Preheat the oven to 375°F (190°C, or gas mark 5) and place the rack in the top third of the oven.

2. Heat the olive oil in a large oven-safe skillet over medium heat. Add the onion and sauté for a few minutes until softened. Then, add the spinach and cook for a few minutes until wilted.

3. Add the bell pepper and mushrooms and continue to sauté for another 2 to 3 minutes until the mushrooms have cooked down and released their moisture.

4. Add the cherry tomatoes, ground cumin, chili powder, garlic powder, salt, and pepper to the skillet. Stir well and continue to sauté for another 2 to 3 minutes.

5. Beat the eggs together in a bowl. Pour the egg mixture over the sautéed vegetables in the skillet and use a spoon to make sure everything is evenly distributed.

6. Place the skillet in the preheated oven and bake for 15 to 20 minutes or until the eggs are set and the top is lightly golden brown.

7. Remove from the oven and let the frittata cool for a few minutes before slicing and serving.

Difficulty: **Easy**

Vegetarian | High Protein | High Fiber | Gluten Free | Grain Free | Nut Free	
Prep Time | 10 minutes	
Cook Time | 20 minutes	
Total Time | 30 minutes	
Yield | 2 servings	
Calories Per Serving | 318	
Total Carbs | 10 g	
Net Carbs | 8 g	
Protein | 21 g	
Fat | 21 g	

Ingredients:

1 tablespoon (28 ml) olive oil

½ small yellow onion, finely diced

1 cup (30 g) spinach, washed and roughly chopped

1 red bell pepper, thinly sliced

½ cup (35 g) white mushrooms, sliced

½ cup (75 g) cherry tomatoes, finely diced

½ teaspoon ground cumin

¼ teaspoon chili powder

¼ teaspoon garlic powder

½ teaspoon salt

¼ teaspoon black pepper

6 large pasture-raised eggs

StrongCurves

Zesty Salmon Power Bowl

As the name suggests, this fresh and zesty power bowl, is a great way to fuel up before your workout. It can be enjoyed warm or cold, so if you're short on time, feel free to prepare it the night before your morning workout.

Instructions:

1. Preheat the oven to 350°F (180°C, or gas mark 5) and place the rack in the middle of the oven.

2. Season the salmon fillet with salt and pepper and place it in the center of a large square piece of parchment paper skin-side up. Make a parcel for the salmon by bringing two sides of the parchment paper together over the fillet and folding them down together, leaving a pocket for the fillet inside. Then, fold the other two sides in to seal the parcel and place on a baking sheet. Bake in the oven for 12 to 15 minutes until cooked through and tender. Remove from the oven and set aside.

3. While the salmon is baking in the oven, cook the quinoa according to package instructions and set aside to cool.

4. In a large bowl, combine the cooled quinoa, avocado, cucumber, red onion, and cherry tomatoes.

5. In a small bowl, whisk together the lime juice, chile flakes, paprika, salt, and pepper.

6. Pour the dressing over the quinoa mixture and toss to combine.

7. Transfer the quinoa into a serving bowl, top with the salmon, and enjoy.

Notes

Please be aware that any ingredient additions, omissions, or substitutions will affect the nutritional information.

- For a keto-friendly option, substitute cauliflower rice for the quinoa.
- If short on cooking time, substitute canned salmon or tuna for the salmon fillet.
- Quinoa can also be bought precooked.
- If making ahead a of time, store the cooked quinoa and salmon fillet separately in the fridge.

Difficulty: **Easy**

High Protein | High Fiber | Pescatarian | Gluten Free | Dairy Free | Egg Free | Nut Free | Keto Friendly (optional)

Prep Time | 10 minutes

Cook Time | 15 minutes

Total Time | 25 minutes

Yield | 1 serving

Calories Per Serving | 449

Total Carbs | 36 g

Net Carbs | 29 g

Protein | 35 g

Fat | 19 g

Ingredients:

4 ounces (115 g) salmon fillet, skin on

½ teaspoon salt, divided

¼ teaspoon black pepper, divided

¼ cup (43 g) quinoa (see notes)

½ avocado, sliced

½ cup (60 g) cucumber, sliced

1 tablespoon (10 g) red onion, finely sliced

¼ cup (38 g) cherry tomatoes, halved

½ lime, juiced

½ teaspoon chile flakes

½ teaspoon smoked paprika

Full English Breakfast Quesadilla

This quesadilla is a healthy twist on the classic full English breakfast, using turkey bacon and fresh ingredients to keep you energized all morning. Enjoy this delicious and easy breakfast before your morning workout or to fuel up for a busy day ahead.

Instructions:

1. In a large nonstick skillet over medium heat, cook the turkey bacon until crispy, about 5 minutes. Remove and set aside.

2. Beat the eggs together in a bowl. Season with salt and pepper and pour into the skillet. Use a spatula to scramble the eggs in the pan until cooked but not overdone.

3. Lay the tortilla on a flat surface. Spoon the scrambled eggs over half of the tortilla. Add the cooked turkey bacon on top of the eggs.

4. Spoon the tomato over the top and sprinkle with cheddar cheese.

5. Fold the other half of the tortilla over the fillings to create a quesadilla.

6. Place the quesadilla in a dry skillet over medium heat and cook for 2 to 3 minutes on each side until the cheese is melted and the tortilla is crispy.

7. Serve hot, garnished with fresh chives.

Difficulty: **Easy**

High Protein | High Fiber | Nut Free

Prep Time | 10 minutes

Cook Time | 15 minutes

Total Time | 25 minutes

Yield | 1 serving

Calories Per Serving | 385

Total Carbs | 19 g

Net Carbs | 17 g

Protein | 26 g

Fat | 22 g

Ingredients:

1 slice of turkey bacon, chopped

2 large pasture-raised eggs

Salt and black pepper, to taste

1 whole wheat or low-carb tortilla (see notes)

¼ cup (45 g) diced tomato

¼ cup (30 g) shredded cheddar cheese

1 tablespoon (3 g) chopped fresh chives

Notes

Please be aware that any ingredient additions, omissions, or substitutions will affect the nutritional information.

- You can use pork bacon in place of turkey bacon, but make sure you use a lean cut and trim the fat before cooking to keep this a high-protein pre-workout option that isn't too high in fat.

- If you prefer a gluten-free or a keto-friendly tortilla substitute, feel free to use a low-carb version such as coconut flour or almond flour tortillas.

StrongCurves

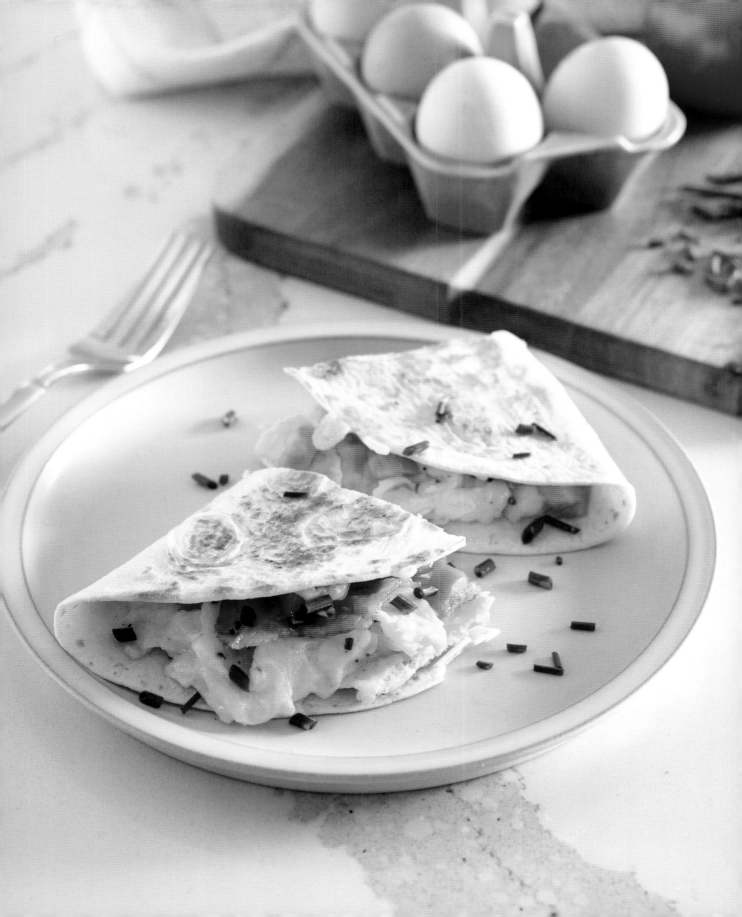

Fuel-Up Breakfast Burger

A healthier version of a fast food favorite, this bun-less breakfast burger is packed with high-protein eggs and bacon, fresh veggies, and a "secret" sauce that's mouth-wateringly good! It's the perfect fuel-up before hitting the gym.

Instructions:

1. Start by making the secret sauce. In a small mixing bowl, add the tomato paste, mayonnaise, mustard, white vinegar, coconut aminos, paprika, garlic powder, onion powder, salt, and pepper. Finely dice half the dill pickle and add it to the mixing bowl. Reserve the other half of the dill pickle for later. Mix the sauce until well combined and set aside.

2. Cook the bacon in a skillet over medium heat until crispy, about 10 minutes. Remove from the skillet and set aside on a paper towel-lined plate.

3. Wipe the skillet clean with a paper towel if needed and return to the stove, lowering the heat if necessary. Crack the eggs into the same skillet and fry to your liking. For over easy eggs, cook until the whites have just set, about 1 to 2 minutes, and then carefully flip them over with a spatula, cooking for another 15 to 30 seconds before removing them from the pan. For over medium eggs, let the whites set and then flip and cook for an additional 30 to 60 seconds.

4. To assemble the burger, layer the lettuce leaves on top of each other on a plate, followed by the tomato, remaining dill pickle, and onion rings. Add the bacon on top of the vegetables, followed by the fried egg. Top with the sauce and then fold the lettuce leaves around the burger.

Notes

When buying store-bought mayonnaise, look for high-quality brands that use olive oil or avocado oil rather than vegetable or seed oils and avoid preservatives and additives. Or use your favorite recipe to make your own homemade mayonnaise!

Difficulty: **Easy**

High Protein | Low Carb | Gluten Free | Dairy Free | Nut Free

Prep Time | 10 minutes

Cook Time | 15 minutes

Total Time | 25 minutes

Yield | 1 serving

Calories Per Serving | 282

Total Carbs | 14 g

Net Carbs | 11 g

Protein | 20 g

Fat | 16 g

Ingredients:

FOR THE BURGERS:

- 3 slices center-cut bacon
- 2 large pasture-raised eggs
- 3–4 iceberg lettuce leaves
- ½ tomato, sliced
- ¼ red onion, sliced into rings

FOR THE SAUCE:

- 1 teaspoon tomato paste
- 1 tablespoon (14 g) olive oil mayonnaise
- ½ teaspoon mustard
- ½ teaspoon white vinegar
- ½ teaspoon coconut aminos or tamari
- ½ teaspoon paprika
- ¼ teaspoon garlic powder
- ¼ teaspoon onion powder
- ¼ teaspoon salt
- ¼ teaspoon black pepper
- 1 small dill pickle

StrongCurves

Vanilla Protein Pudding

This chia pudding is a light and easy breakfast or snack that's high in protein. It's perfect for those who need a quick meal on the go or for those who are looking for a healthy and satisfying dessert.

Instructions:

1. In a bowl, whisk together the almond milk, protein powder, vanilla extract, maple syrup, and sea salt. Add in the chia seeds and whisk until well combined.

2. Cover the bowl with plastic wrap and refrigerate for at least 4 hours or overnight.

3. Once the chia pudding has set, give it a good stir to fluff it up and make sure the chia seeds are evenly distributed.

4. If you prefer a smoother texture, blitz the mixture in a blender for a few minutes, scraping down the sides until you have a creamy and smooth consistency.

5. Divide the chia pudding by spooning it into 2 small mason jars, saving one portion for later. Top with fresh berries. Serve and enjoy!

Notes

Please be aware that any ingredient additions, omissions, or substitutions will affect the nutritional information.

- For a nut-free option, substitute any type of nut-free milk, such as coconut milk, for the almond milk.
- When choosing a protein powder, use a high-quality, clean protein powder from grass-fed cows with no additives, fillers, gums, or anti-caking agents.
- You can also customize the sweetness to your liking by adjusting the amount of maple syrup.
- For a keto-friendly, substitute a few drops of stevia for the maple syrup.

Difficulty: **Easy**

Keto Friendly (optional) | High Protein | Low Carb | Gluten Free | Dairy Free | Egg Free | Nut Free (optional)

Prep Time | 10 minutes

Chill | 4 hours

Total Time | 4 hours, 10 minutes

Yield | 2 servings

Calories Per Serving | 327

Total Carbs | 33 g

Net Carbs | 22 g

Protein | 20 g

Fat | 12 g

Ingredients:

1 cup (235 ml) unsweetened almond milk or nondairy milk of your choice (see notes)

1 scoop vanilla protein powder

1 teaspoon pure vanilla extract

1 tablespoon (15 ml) 100% pure maple syrup (see notes)

Pinch of sea salt

¼ cup (52 g) chia seeds

Fresh berries for topping

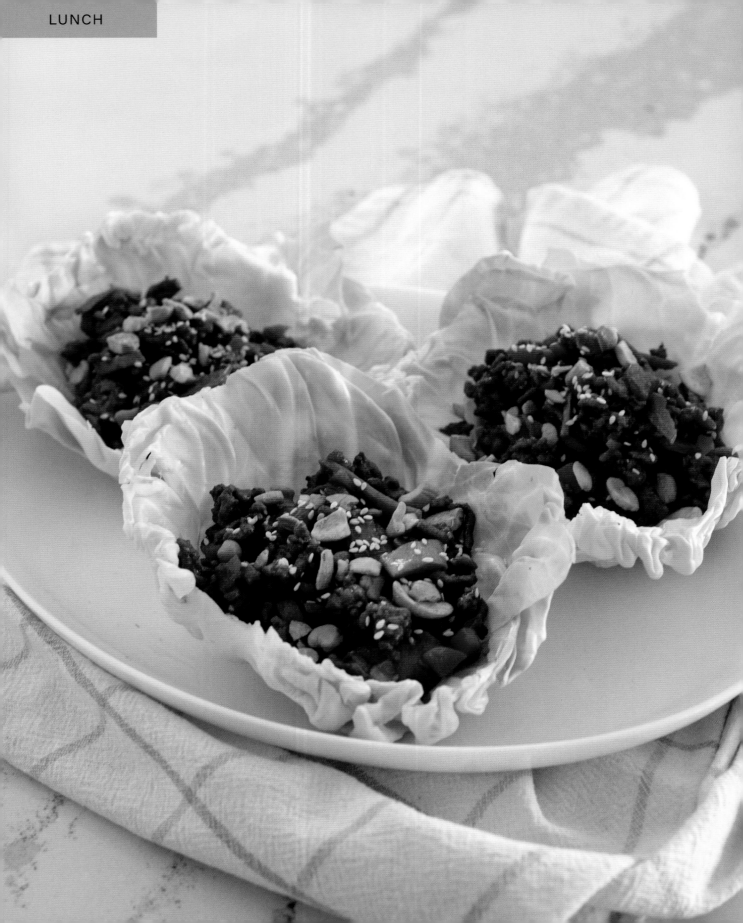

Pork San Choi Bao

This traditional Asian dish, also known as Asian Lettuce Cups or Chinese Lettuce Wraps, is super easy to make and a perfectly light pre-workout meal. The lettuce cups serve as their own little dishes, so you'll be spending less time washing up too. That's a win in my book.

Instructions:

1. In a large skillet, heat the oil over medium heat. Add the onion and carrot and sweat for 5 minutes, stirring regularly, until softened.

2. Add the garlic and ginger and cook for another minute or two until fragrant. Then, add the ground pork, breaking it up with a utensil so that it cooks evenly. Cook the pork until browned, about 3 minutes.

3. Add the bamboo shoots and water chestnuts and stir well. Continue cooking for another 2 to 3 minutes.

4. Add the coconut aminos and arrowroot powder and stir well. Simmer for another 5 minutes until the liquid reduces and sauce thickens slightly.

5. Serve on the lettuce or cabbage leaves. If desired, sprinkle with sesame seeds and cashews. Enjoy!

Difficulty: **Easy**

Dairy Free | Gluten Free | Grain Free | High Protein

Prep Time | 5 minutes

Cook Time | 15 minutes

Total Time | 20 minutes

Yield | 6 servings (12 lettuce cups)

Calories Per Serving | 265

Total Carbs | 13 g

Net Carbs | 10 g

Protein | 37 g

Fat | 8 g

Ingredients:

1 teaspoon coconut or avocado oil

1 small yellow onion, finely diced

1 carrot, finely diced

2 garlic cloves, minced

1 inch (2.5 cm) piece ginger, minced

2 pounds (1 kg) lean ground pork

1 small can (8 ounces, or 225 g) bamboo shoots, drained

1 small can (8 ounces, or 225 g) water chestnuts, drained

¼ cup (60 ml) cup coconut aminos or tamari

1 tablespoon (9 g) arrowroot powder

12 romaine lettuce or green cabbage leaves, washed and trimmed

1 teaspoon sesame seeds (optional)

1 teaspoon crushed raw cashew nuts (optional)

Warm Steak Salad

This recipe pairs juicy beef tenderloin with buttery mushrooms and a refreshing salad for a protein-packed pre-workout lunch.

Instructions:

1. Bring the steak to room temperature ahead of time, letting it rest outside of the fridge for 30 to 40 minutes before cooking. Season it with salt and pepper.

2. Bring a small saucepan of water to a boil and add the green beans. Boil for 3 to 4 minutes until tender and then drain using a sieve. Set aside while you cook the steak.

3. Heat a skillet over high heat and add a bit of oil. Sear the steak for 2 to 3 minutes on each side until a crust forms and then reduce the heat and continue cooking for 4 to 5 minutes on each side until the internal temperature reaches 145°F (63°C) using a meat thermometer. Set aside and let the steak rest.

4. In the same skillet, add a dash more oil and add the garlic, cooking for a minute or so until fragrant. Then, add the mushrooms and cook for another 3 to 5 minutes until they release their liquid and soften. Add the green beans and cook for another 2 to 3 minutes.

5. While the mushrooms and green beans are cooking, prepare the salad by adding the tomato, cucumber, pine nuts, olive oil, coconut aminos, lemon juice, salt, and pepper to a large mixing bowl. Stir to combine.

6. Add the mushroom and green beans to the mixing bowl and stir to combine.

7. Slice the steak into thin strips. Serve the salad onto two plates and top each of them with the sliced steak strips. Enjoy!

Notes

If short on time, make the salad ahead of time and store in an airtight container in the fridge. The steak can also be cooked ahead of time and stored in an airtight container. It won't be warm, but in our opinion it's just as good cold!

Difficulty: Moderate

Dairy Free | Gluten Free | Grain Free | Egg Free | High Protein | High Fiber | Low Carb

Prep Time | 5 minutes

Cook Time | 10 minutes

Total Time | 15 minutes

Yield | 2 servings

Calories Per Serving | 328

Total Carbs | 16 g

Net Carbs | 12 g

Protein | 33 g

Fat | 16 g

Ingredients:

8.8 ounces (246 g) beef tenderloin

½ teaspoon salt, divided

¼ teaspoon black pepper, divided

1 cup (110 g) green beans, trimmed

Olive or avocado oil, for cooking

1 garlic clove, minced

1 cup (70 g) mushrooms, sliced

1 tomato, finely diced

1 cucumber, finely diced

2 teaspoons pine nuts

2 teaspoons olive oil

1 teaspoon coconut aminos or tamari

½ small lemon, juiced

Ham and Egg Cups

These light and fluffy eggs baked in ham slices are a great on-the-go lunch option that can be made ahead of time for an easy and quick high-protein meal when you're dashing out the door on your way to the gym.

Instructions:

1. Preheat the oven to 400°F (200°C, or gas mark 6) and place the rack in the top third of the oven. Grease a muffin pan or line with silicone muffin liners.

2. Beat the eggs together in a mixing bowl. Add the green onion, season with salt and pepper, and give it a good stir to combine.

3. Line the muffin pan with the ham slices, pressing the sides to fit the cup. Pour the egg mixture into the ham cups and top with more green onion and cheddar cheese.

4. Bake for 15 to 20 minutes until the egg is fluffy and golden.

Notes

Please be aware that any ingredient additions, omissions, or substitutions will affect the nutritional information.

- Choose high-quality pasture-raised ham where possible.
- For a dairy-free option, simply omit the shredded cheddar cheese.
- You can enjoy these as a snack at a smaller serving size of 1 to 2 Ham and Egg Cups or as a full meal on their own. They're also delicious served with our Chop-Chop Salad (page 63) or Red Cabbage Slaw (page 64).

Difficulty: **Easy**

Dairy Free (optional) | Gluten Free | Grain Free | High Protein | Low Carb

Prep Time | 5 minutes

Cook Time | 20 minutes

Total Time | 25 minutes

Yield | 3 servings (12 ham and egg cups)

Calories Per Serving | 248

Total Carbs | 12 g

Net Carbs | 8 g

Protein | 21 g

Fat | 12 g

Ingredients:

4 large pasture-raised eggs

1 tablespoon (6 g) chopped green onion, plus more for garnish

½ teaspoon pink Himalayan rock salt

¼ teaspoon black pepper

6 slices ham

¼ cup (30 g) shredded cheddar cheese (optional)

Chicken and Avocado Lettuce Wraps

Packed with protein, fiber, and healthy fats, these wraps make for a light and fresh meal that's perfect as a quick bite before hitting the gym.

Instructions:

1. In a mixing bowl, add the chicken, chili powder, garlic powder, cumin, paprika, salt, and pepper and stir well to combine.

2. In a large skillet, heat the olive oil over medium-high heat. Add the chicken and cook for 8 to 10 minutes or until the chicken is cooked through.

3. While the chicken is cooking, prepare the lettuce leaves by washing and drying them thoroughly. Lay them out on a large plate or serving platter.

4. Once the chicken is cooked through, remove it from the heat and let it cool for a few minutes.

5. To assemble the lettuce wraps, place a few spoonfuls of the cooked chicken in the center of each lettuce leaf. Top with the avocado, tomato, red onion, and cilantro.

6. Squeeze fresh lime juice over the top and then fold the lettuce leaves over the filling to create a wrap. Serve immediately and enjoy!

Notes

For a spicier version, add a dash of cayenne pepper or hot sauce to the chicken while it's cooking.

Difficulty: **Easy**

High Protein | Low Carb | Gluten Free | Dairy Free | Grain Free | Nut Free | Egg Free

Prep Time | 10 minutes

Cook Time | 10 minutes

Total Time | 20 minutes

Yield | 4 servings

Calories Per Serving | 244

Total Carbs | 7 g

Net Carbs | 4 g

Protein | 27 g

Fat | 12 g

Ingredients:

1 pound (466 g) boneless, skinless chicken breasts, diced

¼ teaspoon chili powder

½ teaspoon garlic powder

¼ teaspoon ground cumin

½ teaspoon paprika

½ teaspoon salt

¼ teaspoon black pepper

1 tablespoon (25 ml) olive oil

8 large romaine or iceberg lettuce leaves

1 large avocado, sliced

½ cup (90 g) diced tomato

¼ cup (40 g) finely diced red onion

¼ cup (4 g) chopped fresh cilantro

1 lime, juiced

Egg Salad Wrap

Fuel your body with this delicious take on a lunchtime classic that is packed with protein and healthy fats. It's easy to make and will leave you feeling satisfied and energized.

Instructions:

1. In a small bowl, mix together the hard-boiled eggs, dill pickle, sour cream, Dijon mustard, garlic powder, onion powder, salt, and pepper until well combined.

2. Place the wraps on a flat surface and divide the egg salad mixture between the two wraps. Top each wrap with the turkey bacon. Roll up them up, tucking in the sides as you go, to make a wrap.

3. Serve immediately or store in the refrigerator for up to 2 days.

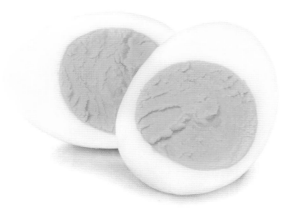

Difficulty: **Easy**

High Protein	Low Carb	Gluten Free	Grain Free	Nut Free	
Prep Time	10 minutes
Total Time	10 minutes
Yield	2 servings
Calories Per Serving	357
Total Carbs	9 g
Net Carbs	7 g
Protein	24 g
Fat	24 g

Ingredients:

5 hard-boiled pasture-raised eggs, chopped

1 dill pickle, finely diced

1 tablespoon (30 g) sour cream

1 tablespoon (5 g) Dijon mustard

¼ teaspoon garlic powder

¼ teaspoon onion powder

¼ teaspoon salt

¼ teaspoon black pepper

2 gluten-free wraps

4 slices turkey bacon, cooked and chopped

Teriyaki Salmon and Bok Choy

This is a simple Asian-inspired dish with flaky melt-in-your-mouth teriyaki salmon. Easily whipped up in under 20 minutes, you can't go wrong with this protein-packed lunch.

Instructions:

1. Preheat the oven to 400°F (200°C, or gas mark 6) and place the rack in the middle of the oven.

2. In a small bowl, make the teriyaki sauce by whisking together the coconut aminos, apple cider vinegar, honey, garlic, and ginger.

3. Season the salmon fillets with salt and pepper on both sides. Place the salmon fillets skin-side down in a baking dish. Pour the teriyaki sauce over the salmon, making sure to coat each fillet evenly.

4. Bake the salmon for 10 to 12 minutes or until it's cooked through and flakes easily with a fork.

5. Meanwhile, heat the olive oil in a large skillet over medium-high heat. Cut the bok choy into quarters and add to the skillet. Season with salt and pepper and sauté for 5 to 7 minutes or until the bok choy is tender and lightly browned.

6. Divide the bok choy among four plates and top with a salmon fillet. Sprinkle with sesame seeds and serve.

Notes

Please be aware that any ingredient additions, omissions, or substitutions will affect the nutritional information.

- To make this recipe spicy, add ¼ teaspoon of chile flakes to the teriyaki sauce.
- You can also substitute another type of fish, such as cod or halibut, for the salmon.

Difficulty: **Easy**

Low Carb	Gluten Free	Dairy Free	Nut Free	Pescatarian	
Prep Time	10 minutes
Cook Time	12 minutes
Total Time	22 minutes
Yield	4 servings
Calories Per Serving	380
Total Carbs	15 g
Net Carbs	14 g
Protein	35 g
Fat	6 g

Ingredients:

- 2 tablespoons (28 ml) coconut aminos or tamari
- 1 tablespoon (15 ml) apple cider vinegar
- 1 tablespoon (20 g) raw honey
- 1 garlic clove, minced
- 1 teaspoon grated fresh ginger
- 4 salmon fillets (6 ounces, or 170 g each), skin on
- ½ teaspoon salt, divided
- ¼ teaspoon black pepper, divided
- 1 tablespoon (28 ml) olive oil
- 4 heads baby bok choy
- 1 tablespoon (8 g) sesame seeds

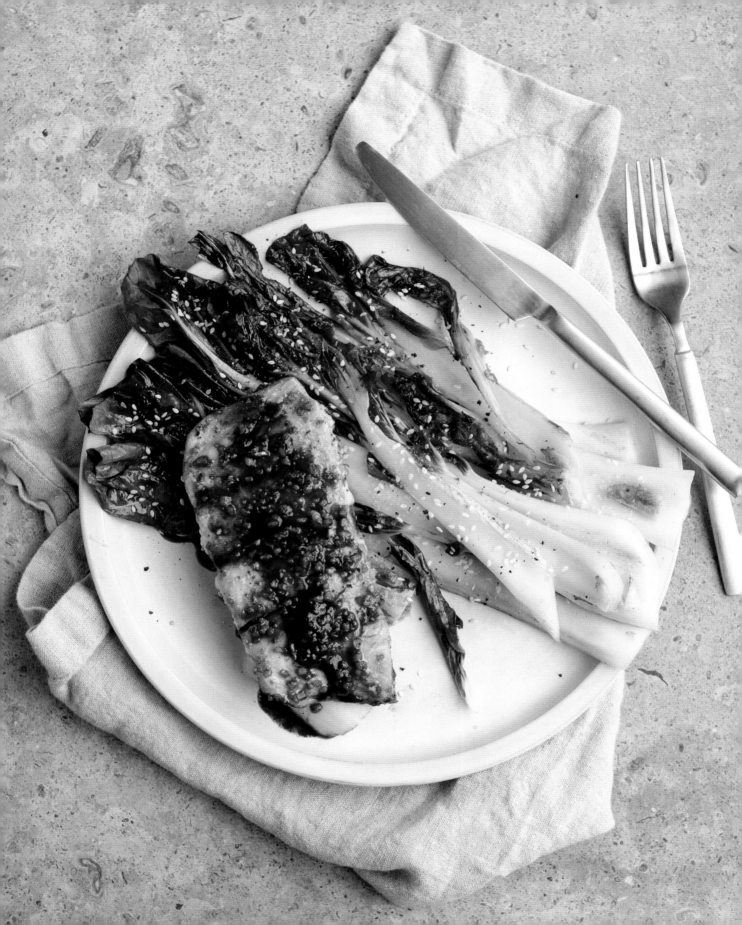

Chicken and Sweet Corn Soup

A comforting family favorite, this chicken and sweet corn soup is a hearty recipe for a pre-workout meal on a cold winter day.

Instructions:

1. Add the bone broth, ginger, and garlic to a large saucepan over medium-high heat.

2. Add the cauliflower and ½ cup (82 g) of the corn to the broth (save the other ½ cup [82 g] for later). Bring to a simmer and cook for 15 minutes or until the cauliflower is soft. Remove from the heat and blend the soup until smooth using an immersion blender. You can also use a standard blender, but you just might have to blend it a few cups at a time.

3. Place the soup back in the saucepan over medium-high heat. Add the remaining ½ cup (82 g) of corn, shredded chicken, and tamari.

4. Stir the arrowroot slurry into the soup. Bring the soup to a gentle simmer and let it simmer until the soup thickens, about 2 to 3 minutes.

5. Use a whisk or a fork to stir the soup, making a slow whirlpool in the center. Slowly drizzle the egg into the whirlpool so that ribbons form in the soup. Season with salt and pepper to taste. Divide among serving bowls and garnish with sliced green onion.

Notes

Please be aware that any ingredient additions, omissions, or substitutions will affect the nutritional information.

- Make the Healing Bone Broth (page 166) ahead of time to use in this recipe. Alternatively, you can buy premade bone broth or stock, but make sure it's from pasture-raised high-quality chicken bones.

- If you prefer a clear and runnier soup, simply omit the arrowroot mixture (also more keto-friendly).

- For a vegetarian option, substitute 1 cup (140 g) of sliced shiitake mushrooms for the chicken and substitute vegetable broth for the chicken bone broth.

Difficulty: **Moderate**

Dairy Free | Gluten Free | Grain Free | High Protein | Low Carb | Nut Free

Prep Time | 10 minutes

Cook Time | 20 minutes

Total Time | 30 minutes

Yield | 2 servings

Calories Per Serving | 367

Total Carbs | 30 g

Net Carbs | 25 g

Protein | 35 g

Fat | 12 g

Ingredients:

4 cups (946 ml) Healing Bone Broth (page 166) or store-bought chicken bone broth (see notes)

1 teaspoon finely grated fresh ginger

2 garlic cloves, crushed

¼ head cauliflower, cut into florets

1 cup (164 g) frozen corn kernels, defrosted or ½ can (15 ounces, or 425 g) corn kernels, drained

1 cup (140 g) shredded chicken, precooked

2 tablespoons (18 g) arrowroot flour, mixed with 2 tablespoons (28 ml) water (optional)

1 pasture-raised egg, beaten

1 tablespoon (15 ml) tamari

Salt and black pepper, to taste

1 tablespoon (6 g) finely sliced green onion, to garnish

StrongCurves

Italian Meatballs

Made with ground pork and ground chicken, these Italian meatballs are tender, juicy, and loaded with veggies in rich tomato sauce. Serve with a side of quinoa, zucchini noodles, or cauliflower rice.

Instructions:

1. In a large mixing bowl, combine the ground pork and chicken, shredded zucchini, spinach, fennel seeds, basil, oregano, garlic, onion powder, chile flakes, salt, and pepper. Mix well with your hands until all the ingredients are combined. Form the mixture into 1-inch (2.5 cm) balls and set aside on a plate.

2. In a large skillet, heat the olive oil over medium heat. Add the meatballs and cook, turning occasionally, until browned on all sides, about 5 to 7 minutes.

3. Reduce the heat to low and add the crushed tomatoes to the skillet. Cover the skillet and simmer for 10 to 15 minutes until the meatballs are cooked through. Serve hot and garnish with parsley.

Notes

Please be aware that any ingredient additions, omissions, or substitutions will affect the nutritional information.

- Pork and chicken work best in this recipe as they tend to stay more tender and moist compared to beef. If you prefer, you can use only ground chicken instead of the pork/chicken mix. Make sure to use pasture-raised and high-quality pork or chicken.

- Made in bulk, you can store these meatballs in the fridge for up to 5 days and also freeze them for later use.

Difficulty: **Easy**

High Protein | Low Carb | Gluten Free | Dairy Free | Nut Free

Prep Time | 10 minutes

Cook Time | 30 minutes

Total Time | 40 minutes

Yield | 4 servings (20 meatballs)

Calories Per Serving | 397

Total Carbs | 4 g

Net Carbs | 3 g

Protein | 31 g

Fat | 28 g

Ingredients:

¾ pound (340 g) lean ground pork

¾ pound (340 g) ground chicken

1 cup (120 g) shredded zucchini

1 cup (30 g) finely chopped spinach

½ teaspoon fennel seeds

½ teaspoon dried basil

½ teaspoon dried oregano

2 cloves garlic, minced

½ teaspoon onion powder

¼ teaspoon chile flakes

½ teaspoon salt

¼ teaspoon black pepper

1 tablespoon (28 ml) olive oil (for frying)

1 can (14 ounces, or 390 g) crushed tomatoes

1 tablespoon (4 g) chopped fresh parsley, to garnish

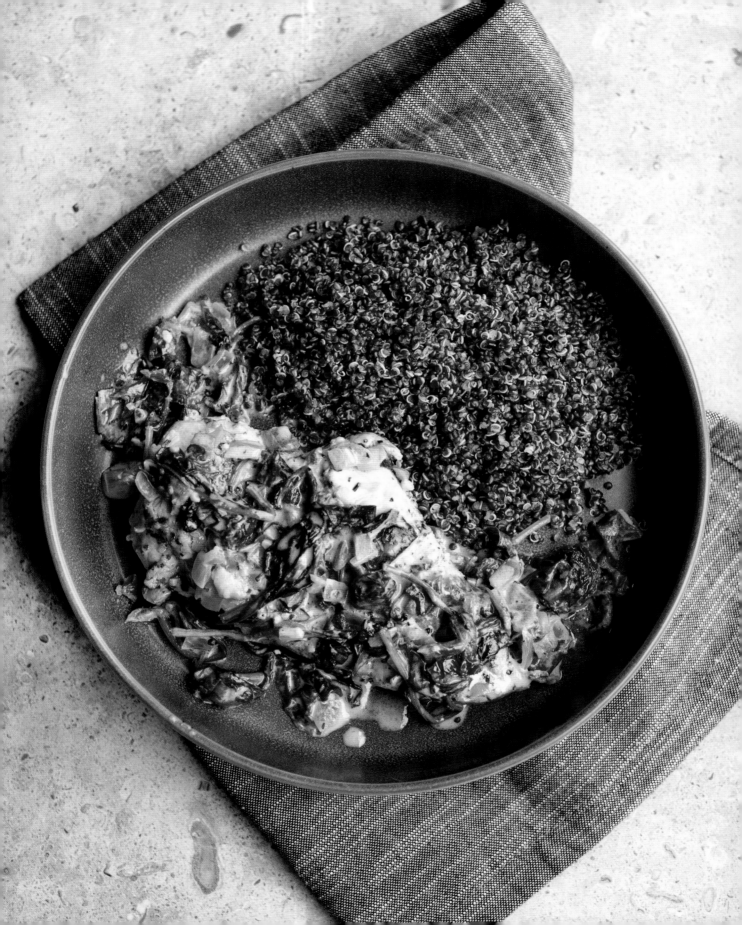

Creamy Tuscan Chicken

This dairy-free Creamy Tuscan Chicken uses coconut cream and fragrant herbs to create a luscious, velvety sauce that complements the tender chicken perfectly. It's a great midweek dinner option before your late night gym session . . . and the leftovers are almost even better.

Instructions:

1. In a small mixing bowl, add the thyme, oregano, salt, pepper, and chile flakes and mix well. If the chicken breasts are rather large, place them between two pieces of parchment paper and pound them down to make them thinner or butterfly them using a sharp knife. Transfer the chicken breasts to a plate and sprinkle both sides with the herb and spice mix.

2. Add the oil to a large skillet over medium-high heat. Add the chicken and cook for 4 to 5 minutes on each side until browned and nearly cooked through. Remove the chicken from the skillet and set aside.

3. In the same skillet, add the onion and garlic. Sauté until the onion is soft and translucent, about 3 to 4 minutes.

4. Pour in the chicken bone broth and coconut milk and stir until well combined. Add the sun-dried tomatoes and stir to incorporate.

5. Reduce the heat to low and add the baby spinach to the skillet. Stir until the spinach has wilted and the sauce has thickened, about 2 to 3 minutes.

6. Return the chicken to the skillet and spoon the sauce over the chicken. Cover the skillet and simmer for another 5 to 7 minutes until the sauce is thick and creamy and the chicken registers an internal temperature of 165°F (75°C).

7. Serve hot with a side of your choice such as zucchini noodles, quinoa, or cauliflower rice.

Notes

Make the Healing Bone Broth (page 166) ahead of time to use in this recipe. Alternatively, you can buy premade bone broth or stock, but make sure it's from pasture-raised high-quality chicken bones.

Difficulty: **Easy**

High Protein | Low Carb| Dairy Free | Gluten Free | Grain Free | Nut Free | Egg Free

Prep Time | 10 minutes

Cook Time | 20 minutes

Total Time | 30 minutes

Yield | 4 servings

Calories Per Serving | 341

Total Carbs | 28 g

Net Carbs | 26 g

Protein | 29 g

Fat | 13 g

Ingredients:

1 teaspoon dried thyme

1 teaspoon dried oregano

½ teaspoon salt

¼ teaspoon black pepper

¼ teaspoon chile flakes

4 boneless, skinless chicken breasts

1 tablespoon (28 ml) avocado or olive oil

1 onion, diced

2 cloves garlic, minced

½ cup (120 ml) Healing Bone Broth (page 166) or store-bought chicken bone broth (see notes)

½ cup (120 ml) canned coconut milk

½ cup (28 g) sun-dried tomatoes, chopped

2 cups (86 g) baby spinach

Chicken Shish Taouk Skewers

Here's a high-protein Middle Eastern chicken dish that's juicy, tender, and packed full of flavor. Enjoy with a side salad or cauliflower rice for a pre-workout meal. It's also great served with couscous or steamed rice as a post-workout meal.

Instructions:

1. In a small mixing bowl, add the yogurt, olive oil, lemon juice, tomato paste, garlic, spices, salt, and pepper and mix well until combined. Add the chicken to the yogurt marinade, mixing thoroughly. Let chill in the fridge for at least 4 hours.

2. Remove from the fridge and thread the chicken pieces onto metal skewers. (You can use wooden skewers too. Just be sure to soak them beforehand for 30 minutes so they don't splinter.)

3. Heat a griddle pan over medium-high heat and cook chicken skewers for 10 minutes or until cooked through, turning the skewers every couple minutes to allow even cooking.

4. Remove from the heat and serve with Chop-Chop Salad (page 63) or Red Cabbage Slaw (page 64).

Difficulty: **Easy**

High Protein | Low Carb | Gluten Free | Grain Free | Nut Free | Egg Free

Prep Time | 10 minutes

Chill Time | 4 hours

Cook Time | 10 minutes

Total Time | 4 hours 20 minutes

Yield | 6 servings

Calories Per Serving | 241

Total Carbs | 3 g

Net Carbs | 2 g

Protein | 40 g

Fat | 11 g

Ingredients:

½ cup (115 g) full-fat natural yogurt

¼ cup (60 ml) olive oil

1 tablespoon (15 ml) lemon juice

1 tablespoon (16 g) tomato paste

1 garlic clove, minced

1 teaspoon dried oregano

1 teaspoon smoked paprika

½ teaspoon ground ginger

½ teaspoon ground cumin

¼ teaspoon ground cinnamon

1 teaspoon salt

¼ teaspoon black pepper

28 ounces (795 g) skinless, boneless chicken breast, diced into 1 inch (2.5 cm) cubes

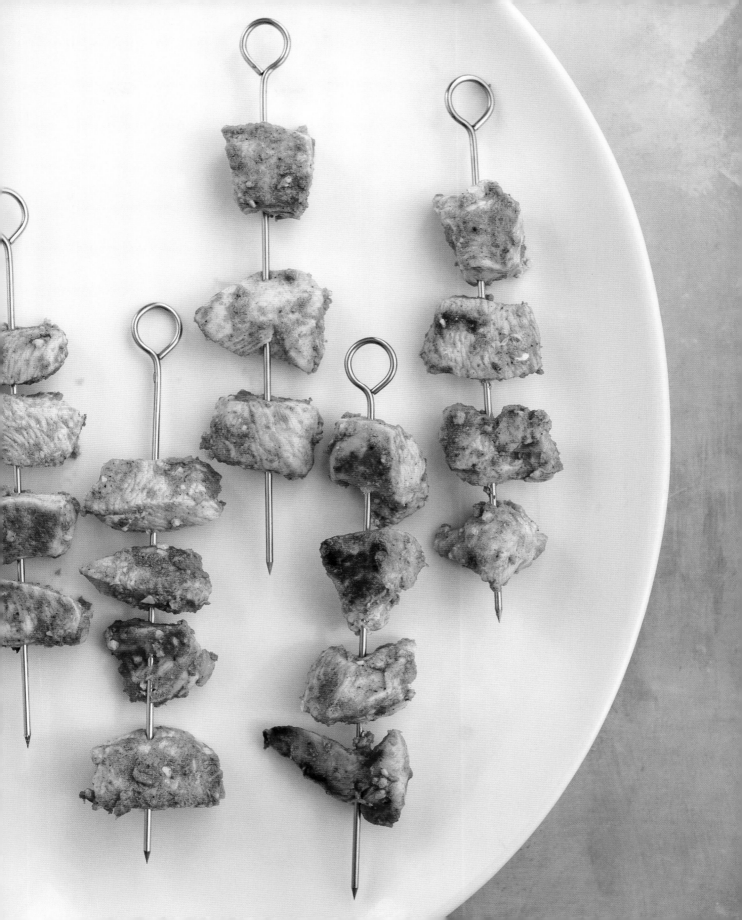

Stuffed Cabbage Rolls

A simple and satisfying casserole that the whole family will love, this dish features Italian-style ground beef wrapped into rolls and baked in a rich tomato sauce.

Instructions:

1. Bring a large pot of water to a boil and add the cabbage leaves. Bring the heat down to a simmer, cover with a lid, and cook for 2 to 3 minutes until the leaves have softened. Remove from the pot and set aside for later.

2. Preheat the oven to 350°F (180°C, or gas mark 4) and place a rack in the center of the oven.

3. Add the onion and garlic to a large skillet over medium heat and sauté until soft and translucent, about 2 to 3 minutes. Add the ground beef and stir, breaking it down with a wooden spoon so that it browns evenly. Drain any excess fat. Add the cauliflower rice, parsley, and Italian seasoning and cook for 3 to 4 minutes.

4. Combine the tomato purée and tomato paste in a small bowl. Pour a third of this mixture into the beef mixture, reserving the rest for later. Stir to combine and cook for another 2 to 3 minutes.

5. In a casserole dish, spread a thin layer of the reserved tomato sauce on the bottom of the dish (about 1 tablespoon [15 ml]).

6. Cut the stems out of the cabbage leaves and fill each leaf with ⅓ cup (80 ml) of the beef mixture. Roll the cabbage lengthwise (like a cigar), tucking the sides in, and place seam-side down in the dish. Repeat for all the cabbage leaves.

7. Top the cabbage rolls with the remaining tomato sauce and cheddar cheese. Bake for 60 to 75 minutes until the cheese is golden and the cabbage rolls are tender.

Notes

Please be aware that any ingredient additions, omissions, or substitutions will affect the nutritional information.

- Ground turkey, chicken, or pork also works well in this recipe..
- For a dairy-free option, simply omit the cheddar cheese.

Difficulty: **Moderate**

High Protein | Strict Low Carb | Gluten Free | Grain Free | Egg Free | Nut Free | Dairy Free (optional)

Prep Time | 20 minutes

Cook Time | 1 hour, 15 minutes

Total Time | 1 hour, 35 minutes

Yield | 5 servings

Calories Per Serving | 427

Total Carbs | 13 g

Net Carbs | 11 g

Protein | 43 g

Fat | 24 g

Ingredients:

10 cabbage leaves

1 yellow onion, diced

1 garlic clove, minced

2 pounds (900 g) lean ground beef

2 cups (200 g) cauliflower (½ head), grated or processed in a food processor

2 tablespoons (8 g) chopped fresh parsley

1 tablespoon (6 g) Italian seasoning

1 cup (250 g) tomato purée

2 tablespoons (32 g) tomato paste

½ cup (58 g) shredded cheddar cheese (optional)

Strong*Curves*

Tuna Casserole

This twist on an American classic might not feature noodles as the typical carb-heavy version does, but it's packed with protein and healthy Omega-3 fatty acids for an awesome energy boost before your workout. Made with canned tuna and a creamy sauce, this is a dish that the whole family will love. I promise you won't even notice the missing noodles.

Instructions:

1. Preheat the oven to 350°F (180°C, or gas mark 4).

2. In a large mixing bowl, combine the tuna, mayonnaise, Dijon mustard, sour cream, half of the Gruyère cheese (reserve the other half), red onion, parsley, lemon juice, garlic powder, paprika, salt, and pepper. Stir until well combined.

3. Transfer the mixture to a casserole dish and spread it evenly. Sprinkle the remaining cheese on top.

4. Bake in the oven for 15 to 20 minutes until the top is golden and bubbly.

5. Let the casserole cool for a few minutes before serving.

Notes

Please be aware that any ingredient additions, omissions, or substitutions will affect the nutritional information.

- When choosing store-bought canned tuna, choose wild-caught tuna in brine, not oil.
- When buying store-bought mayonnaise, look for high-quality brands that use olive oil or avocado oil rather than vegetable or seed oils and avoid preservatives and additives. Or use your favorite recipe to make your own homemade mayonnaise!
- For a dairy-free option, omit the sour cream and Gruyère cheese.
- Leftovers can be stored in the fridge for up to 3 days.

Difficulty: **Easy**

High Protein | Pescatarian | Low Carb | Gluten Free | Nut Free | Dairy Free (optional)	
Prep Time | 10 minutes	
Cook Time | 20 minutes	
Total Time | 35 minutes	
Yield | 4 servings	
Calories Per Serving | 412	
Total Carbs | 7 g	
Net Carbs | 7 g	
Protein | 36 g	
Fat | 26 g	

Ingredients:

4 cans (5 ounces, or 140 g each) tuna in water, drained

⅔ cup (150 g) olive oil mayonnaise

2 tablespoons (10 g) Dijon mustard

½ cup (115 g) sour cream (optional)

½ cup (60 g) shredded Gruyère cheese (optional)

¼ (40 g) red onion, finely chopped

2 tablespoons (8 g) chopped fresh parsley

1 tablespoon (15 ml) lemon juice

1 teaspoon garlic powder

½ teaspoon paprika

½ teaspoon salt

¼ teaspoon black pepper

Grilled Shrimp and Zucchini Salad

This refreshing salad combines grilled shrimp with fresh and crispy greens in a zesty lemon dressing, giving you everything you need before your workout: protein, healthy fats, and fiber.

Instructions:

1. Heat a little olive oil on a grill pan or skillet over medium-high heat.

2. Add the shrimp to the grill pan or skillet and cook for 2 to 3 minutes on each side until cooked through. Set aside. Now add the zucchini to the same pan, laying each piece flat and cook for 2 to 3 minutes on each side until softened and charred. Be careful not to overcrowd the pan—you may need to cook the zucchini in two batches.

3. To make the dressing, whisk together the olive oil, lemon juice, Dijon mustard, garlic, salt, and pepper in a small mixing bowl.

4. In a large mixing bowl, combine the mixed greens, cherry tomatoes, red onion, and basil.

5. Add the grilled shrimp and zucchini to the mixing bowl and toss to combine.

6. Drizzle the lemon dressing over the salad and toss to coat.

Notes

This salad can be made ahead of time and stored in the fridge for up to 2 days. Just wait to add the dressing until right before serving to prevent the greens from wilting.

Difficulty: **Easy**

High Protein | Pescatarian | Low Carb | Gluten Free | Nut Free | Dairy Free | Egg Free

Prep Time | 10 minutes

Cook Time | 10 minutes

Total Time | 20 minutes

Yield | 2 servings

Calories Per Serving | 261

Total Carbs | 8 g

Net Carbs | 5 g

Protein | 27 g

Fat | 14 g

Ingredients:

2 tablespoons (28 ml) olive oil, plus more for cooking

10 medium-sized shrimp, peeled and deveined

1 medium-sized zucchini, sliced into thin ribbons

1 tablespoon (15 ml) lemon juice

1 teaspoon Dijon mustard

1 garlic clove, minced

Salt and black pepper, to taste

4 cups (220 g) mixed greens

¼ cup (38 g) cherry tomatoes, halved

1 tablespoon (10 g) red onion, finely diced

¼ cup (4 g) fresh basil leaves, chopped

StrongCurves

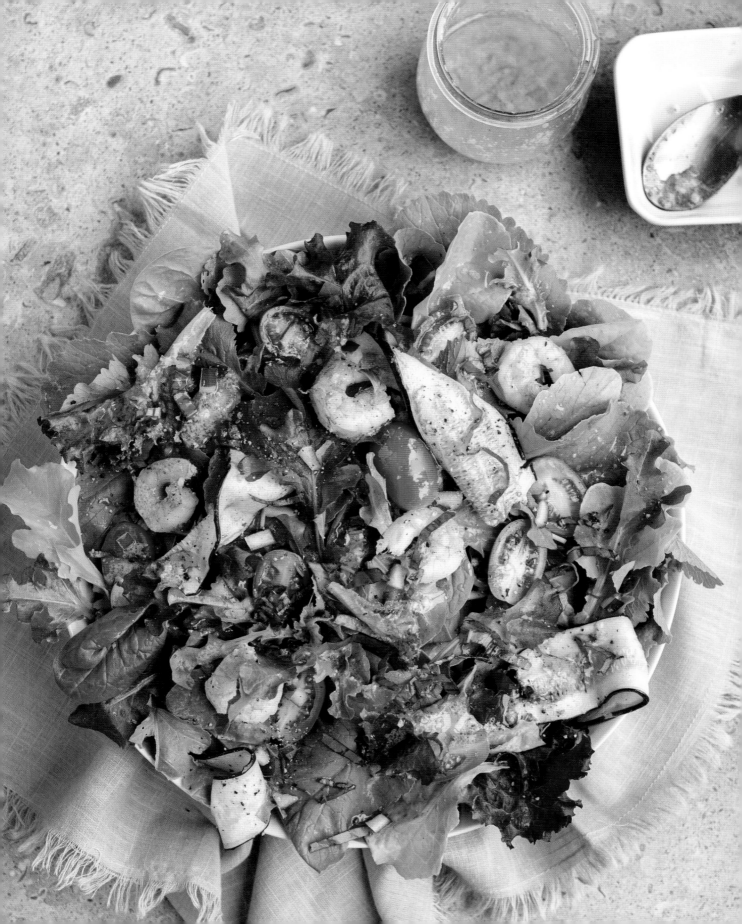

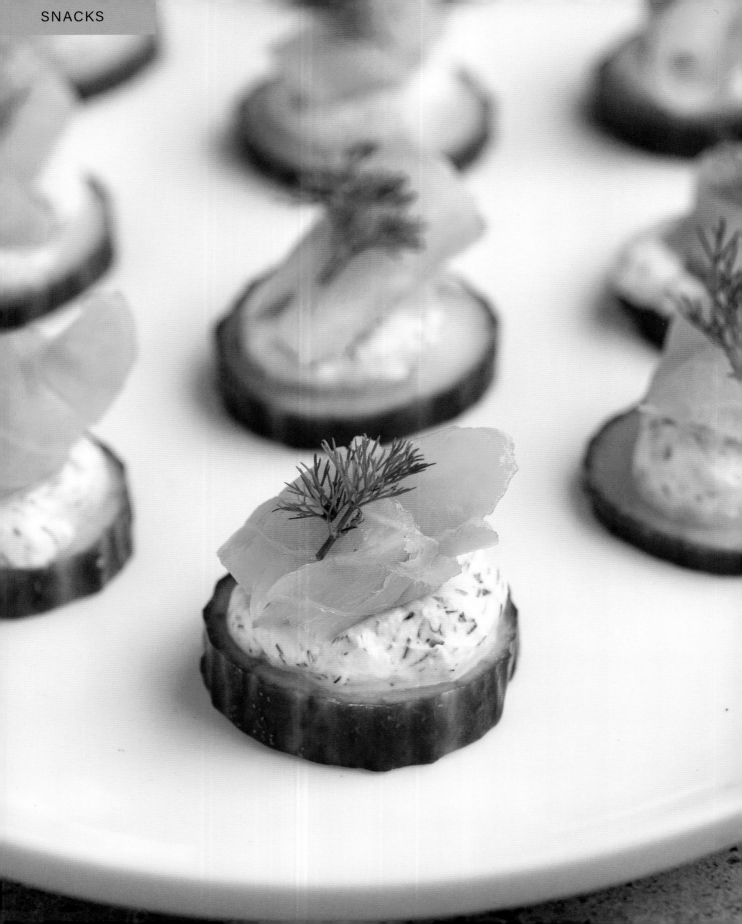

Salmon and Cucumber Canapés

These refreshingly light canapés feature smoked salmon, dill, and cream cheese for a perfect pre-workout snack or as an appetizer that's sure to be a crowd pleaser.

Instructions:

1. In a small bowl, mix together the cream cheese, dill, and lemon juice until well combined. Season with salt and pepper to taste.

2. Lay out the cucumber slices on a platter or serving dish. Top each cucumber slice with a small dollop of the cream cheese mixture. Fold a slice of smoked salmon into a small roll and place it on top of the cream cheese mixture. Garnish each canapé with a small sprig of fresh dill.

3. Serve immediately or refrigerate until ready to use.

Notes

Please be aware that any ingredient additions, omissions, or substitutions will affect the nutritional information.

- For a creamier texture, you can also blend the cream cheese mixture along with the salmon in a food processor or blender until smooth.
- You can also substitute cooked salmon or other types of smoked fish, such as trout or mackerel, for the smoked salmon.

Difficulty: **Easy**

High Protein | Low Carb | Pescatarian | Gluten Free | Nut Free | Egg Free

Prep Time | 10 minutes

Total Time | 10 minutes

Yield | 5 servings (10 canapés)

Calories Per Serving | 81

Total Carbs | 2 g

Net Carbs | 2 g

Protein | 9 g

Fat | 4 g

Ingredients:

2 tablespoons (30 g) dairy-free cream cheese

1 tablespoon (4 g) chopped fresh dill

1 tablespoon (15 ml) lemon juice

Salt and pepper, to taste

10 slices cucumber, about ¼-inch (6 mm) thick

½ pound (225 g) smoked salmon

Greek Yogurt and Berries

This creamy and naturally sweet snack provides a good source of protein, healthy fats, fiber, and antioxidants.

Instructions:

1. In a medium bowl, mix together the yogurt, honey, and vanilla extract until well combined.

2. Wash the berries and slice any large ones into bite-sized pieces. Add the berries to the yogurt mixture and gently stir to combine.

3. Divide the mixture into two bowls and sprinkle with the chopped walnuts. Serve immediately or chill in the fridge for later.

Notes

Please be aware that any ingredient additions, omissions, or substitutions will affect the nutritional information.

- For a dairy-free option, substitute coconut yogurt for the Greek yogurt.
- For a keto-friendly option, substitute a keto-friendly sweetener, such as stevia, monk fruit, or erythritol, for the honey.
- Other nuts such as almonds or pecans also work well in this recipe.

Difficulty: **Easy**

Low Carb | Gluten Free | Grain Free | Vegetarian | Egg Free | Dairy Free (optional) | Keto Friendly (optional)

Prep Time | 5 minutes

Total Time | 5 minutes

Yield | 2 servings

Calories Per Serving | 160

Total Carbs | 17 g

Net Carbs | 16 g

Protein | 6 g

Fat | 8 g

Ingredients:

1 cup (230 g) natural full-fat Greek yogurt (see notes)

2 teaspoons raw honey (see notes)

¼ teaspoon pure vanilla extract (optional)

½ cup (70 g) mixed berries (such as strawberries, blueberries, and raspberries)

2 tablespoons (15 g) chopped walnuts

Protein Bento Box

This bento box is a quick and easy no-cook snack that packs a protein punch, keeping you energized and ready to smash your workout even if it's been a while between meals.

Instructions:

1. Start by arranging a bento box or a similar container with dividers. Add the turkey breast to one of the compartments. In a separate compartment, add the hard-boiled egg. In another compartment, add cherry tomatoes and cucumber. In the remaining compartment, add the olives and feta cheese. In a separate small container, add the hummus. Cover the bento box and refrigerate until ready to eat.

Notes

Please be aware that any ingredient additions, omissions, or substitutions will affect the nutritional information.

Feel free to swap out the protein sources with your favorites, such as grilled salmon or chicken.

Difficulty: **Easy**

High Protein | Low Carb | Gluten Free | Grain Free | Nut Free

Prep Time | 10 minutes

Total Time | 10 minutes

Yield | 1 serving

Calories Per Serving | 346

Total Carbs | 13 g

Net Carbs | 10 g

Protein | 37 g

Fat | 16 g

Ingredients:

3 ounces (85 g) sliced turkey breast

1 hard-boiled pasture-raised egg, peeled

½ cup (75 g) cherry tomatoes

½ cup (60 g) sliced cucumber

5 pitted black olives

1 ounce (28 g) feta cheese, cubed

1 tablespoon (15 g) hummus

Blueberry and Zucchini Muffins

These blueberry and zucchini muffins are moist, light, and just the right amount of sweet. They're packed with fresh blueberries and shredded zucchini, making them high in fiber—a perfect workout-friendly snack.

Instructions:

1. Preheat the oven to 350°F (180°C, or gas mark 4) and place the rack in the middle of the oven. Grease a muffin pan or line with silicone muffin liners.

2. In a medium bowl, whisk together the almond flour, baking powder, and salt.

3. In a separate bowl, beat together the coconut oil, coconut sugar, lemon juice, lemon zest, eggs, and vanilla extract until well combined.

4. Add the dry ingredients to the wet mixture and stir until just combined.

5. Fold in the shredded zucchini and fresh blueberries.

6. Divide the batter evenly between the muffin cups.

7. Bake for 20 to 25 minutes or until a toothpick comes out clean. Allow the muffins to cool in the pan for 5 minutes before transferring them to a wire rack to cool completely.

Notes

Please be aware that any ingredient additions, omissions, or substitutions will affect the nutritional information.

- To strain the zucchini, use a cheesecloth to squeeze as much of the liquid out of the veggies as possible; otherwise, the muffins will turn out soggy.
- For a keto-friendly option, use erythritol or any other granulated sweetener of your choice in place of the coconut sugar.
- Store the muffins in an airtight container at room temperature for up to 3 days or in the fridge for up to a week. They can also be frozen for longer storage.

Difficulty: **Easy**

Low Carb | Gluten Free | Grain Free | Dairy Free | Vegetarian | Keto Friendly (optional)	
Prep Time | 10 minutes	
Cook Time | 25 minutes	
Total Time | 35 minutes	
Yield | 12 muffins	
Calories Per Muffin | 226	
Total Carbs | 11 g	
Net Carbs | 8 g	
Protein | 6 g	
Fat | 20 g	

Ingredients:

2 cups (224 g) blanched almond flour

2 teaspoons baking powder

¼ teaspoon salt

½ cup (112 g) coconut oil, melted

¼ cup (36 g) coconut sugar (see notes)

1 tablespoon (15 ml) lemon juice

1 tablespoon (6 g) lemon zest

3 large pasture-raised eggs

1 teaspoon pure vanilla extract

1½ cups (180 g) shredded zucchini, strained (see notes)

1 cup (145 g) fresh blueberries

StrongCurves

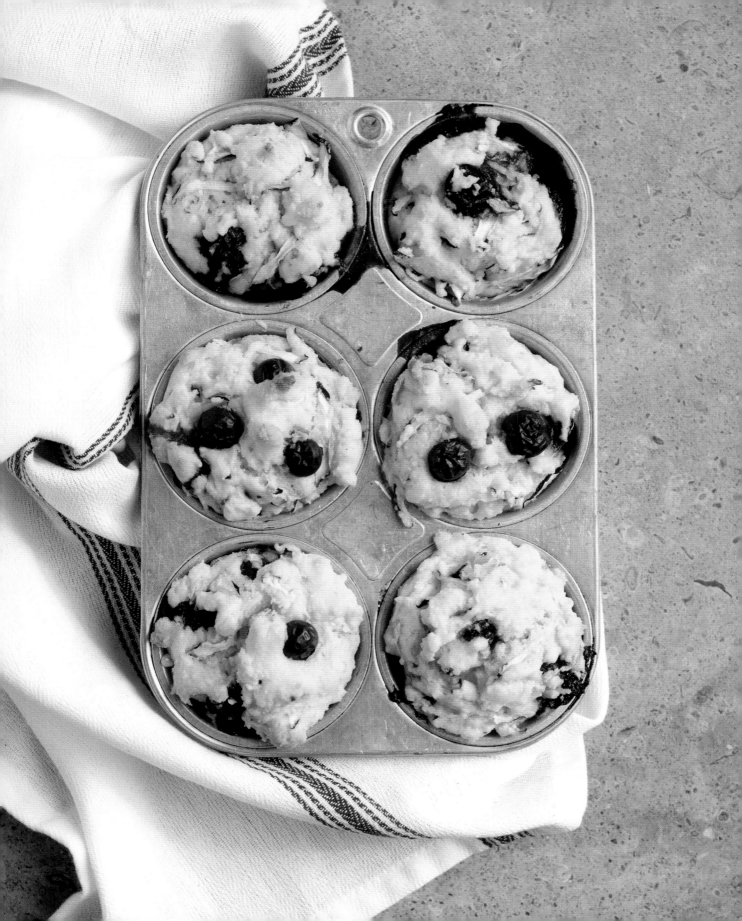

Chewy Fig Protein Bar

Skip the store-bought energy bars. These homemade fiber-packed fig bars are chewy, chocolatey, packed with protein, and just the right amount of sweet.

Instructions:

1. Preheat the oven to 350°F (180°C, or gas mark 4) and place the rack in the middle of the oven. Line an 8 x 8-inch (20 x 20-cm) baking pan with parchment paper.

2. In a large mixing bowl, combine the almond flour, cinnamon, and salt. Mix until well combined. In a separate bowl, whisk together the coconut oil, coconut sugar, and vanilla extract until smooth. Pour the wet mixture over the dry mixture and stir until a soft dough forms. Press the dough evenly into the pan and bake for 15 to 20 minutes until golden and cooked through. Set aside and let cool.

3. While the crust is baking, combine the dried figs, water, and orange juice in a small saucepan on a low heat. Cover and simmer for 8 to 10 minutes or until the figs plump up and the sauce thickens. Remove from the heat and set aside to cool.

4. Transfer the fig mixture to a food processor. Add the honey, shredded coconut, and protein powder and blend until a thick paste forms. Transfer the mixture to the prepared baking pan and spread it out evenly on top of the crust.

5. To make the chocolate topping, add the chocolate chips to a heat-proof bowl over a small saucepan of simmering water on a low heat, stirring often with a spoon or spatula. When the chocolate is fully melted, remove from the heat.

6. Spread the melted chocolate on top of the fig filling, top with chopped nuts, and chill in the fridge for a minimum of 2 hours. Once they've set, remove them from the fridge, slice into 12 bars, and serve immediately or keep in an airtight container in the fridge for later.

Difficulty: **Easy**

Low Carb | Vegetarian | Gluten Free | Grain Free | Egg Free

Prep Time | 15 minutes

Cook Time | 20 minutes

Chill Time | 2 hours

Total Time | 2 hours, 35 minutes

Yield | 14 bars

Calories Per Bar | 215

Total Carbs | 16 g

Net Carbs | 13 g

Protein | 9 g

Fat | 13 g

Ingredients:

FOR THE CRUST:

½ cup (56 g) almond flour

½ teaspoon ground cinnamon

¼ teaspoon salt

¼ cup (55 g) coconut oil, melted

¼ cup (36 g) coconut sugar

1 teaspoon pure vanilla extract

FOR THE FIG FILLING:

1 cup (150 g) dried figs, chopped

½ cup (120 ml) water (or more as needed)

2 tablespoons (28 ml) 100% pure fresh orange juice

2 teaspoons raw honey

¼ cup (20 g) unsweetened shredded coconut

4 scoops protein powder

FOR THE CHOCOLATE TOPPING:

⅓ cup (80 g) unsweetened dark chocolate chips

¼ cup (36 g) mixed raw nuts, roughly chopped

Chop-Chop Salad

This is a fresh mix of diced cucumber and juicy cherry tomatoes in a simple salad dressing.

Instructions:

1. Combine the cherry tomatoes and cucumber in a salad bowl. Add the rest of the ingredients and stir well to combine. Serve and enjoy!

Notes

Serve as a side to Chicken Shish Taouk Skewers (page 50).

Difficulty: **Easy**

Low Carb | Gluten Free | Grain Free | Dairy Free | Egg Free | Nut Free | Vegetarian

Prep Time	5 minutes
Total Time	5 minutes
Yield	2 servings
Calories Per Serving	76
Total Carbs	10 g
Net Carbs	8 g
Protein	2 g
Fat	5 g

Ingredients:

6 cherry tomatoes, finely diced

1 large cucumber, finely diced

1 teaspoon coconut aminos or tamari

2 teaspoons olive oil

½ lemon, juiced

¼ teaspoon salt

¼ teaspoon black pepper

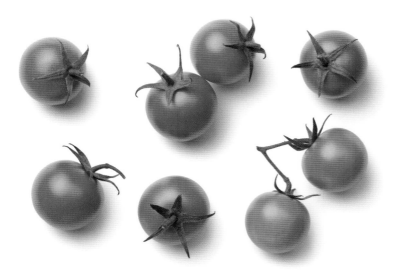

Red Cabbage Slaw

A crunchy and creamy slaw of red cabbage, carrots, and fragrant cumin, this high-fiber side salad is full of healthy fats and goes perfectly with any main meat dish.

Instructions:

1. Add the red cabbage and carrot to a large salad bowl and toss to combine.

2. Add the sunflower seeds, pepitas, lemon juice, mayonnaise, parsley, cumin, salt, and pepper and toss to fully incorporate. Serve and enjoy!

Notes

- When buying store-bought mayonnaise, look for high-quality brands that use olive oil or avocado oil rather than vegetable or seed oils and avoid preservatives and additives. Or use your favorite recipe to make your own homemade mayonnaise!

- Serve as a side to Chicken Shish Taouk Skewers (page 50) or Italian Meatballs (page 47)

Difficulty: **Easy**

Low Carb | Gluten Free | Grain Free | Dairy Free | Vegetarian

Prep Time | 5 minutes

Total Time | 5 minutes

Yield | 2 servings

Calories Per Serving | 110

Total Carbs | 10 g

Net Carbs | 7 g

Protein | 3 g

Fat | 7 g

Ingredients:

1½ cups (105 g) shredded red cabbage

½ cup (55 g) shredded carrot

1 tablespoon (9 g) sunflower seeds

1 tablespoon (9 g) pepitas

½ lemon, juiced

1 tablespoon (14 g) olive oil mayonnaise

1 tablespoon (4 g) chopped fresh parsley

¼ teaspoon ground cumin

½ teaspoon salt

¼ teaspoon black pepper

Sautéed Green Beans and Mushrooms

Garlic sautéed green beans and buttery mushrooms make this a go-to side with any main dish.

Instructions:

1. Bring a saucepan of water to boil. Add the green beans and lower the heat. Simmer for 2 to 3 minutes until beans are tender but still crunchy. Remove from the heat, drain, and set aside.

2. Add a little butter to a skillet over medium heat. Add the garlic to the pan and sauté for 1 to 2 minutes until fragrant.

3. Add the mushrooms to the pan. Sauté for 3 to 5 minutes until the mushrooms break down and release their liquid. Add the pine nuts and green beans and cook for a few minutes, stirring occasionally. Season with salt and pepper. Serve and enjoy!

Notes

Please be aware that any ingredient additions, omissions, or substitutions will affect the nutritional information.

- For a dairy-free option, substitute coconut oil for the grass-fed butter.
- Serve as a side to Chicken Shish Taouk Skewers (page 50) or Italian Meatballs (page 47).

Difficulty: **Easy**

Low Carb | Gluten Free | Grain Free | Dairy Free (optional) | Egg Free | Vegetarian

Prep Time	5 minutes
Cook Time	10 minutes
Total Time	15 minutes
Yield	2 servings
Calories Per Serving	59
Total Carbs	9 g
Net Carbs	6 g
Protein	3 g
Fat	2 g

Ingredients:

2 cups (220 g) green beans, trimmed and sliced

1 teaspoon grass-fed butter (see notes)

1 garlic clove, minced

5 button mushrooms, sliced

1 tablespoon (18 g) pine nuts

½ teaspoon salt

¼ teaspoon black pepper

Cheesy Broccoli Poppers

These broccoli poppers are extra cheesy with just the right amount of spice. Easy finger food, they're sure to be a hit at any gathering or as a quick grab and go snack. Enjoy them hot or cold!

Instructions:

1. Preheat the oven to 375°F (190°C, or gas mark 5).

2. In a large mixing bowl, combine the broccoli, cheddar cheese, almond flour, garlic, onion powder, chile flakes, paprika, salt, and pepper. Mix well to combine.

3. Add the beaten eggs to the mixture and stir until all ingredients are well combined.

4. Using a small cookie scoop or spoon, form the mixture into small balls about 1 inch (2.5 cm) in diameter.

5. Place them on a baking sheet lined with parchment paper and bake for 15 to 20 minutes until golden brown and cooked through.

6. Remove from the oven and let cool slightly on a wire rack before serving.

Notes

- Make sure to finely dice the broccoli florets to ensure they cook evenly and are easy to form into poppers. Alternatively, you can blend them in a food processor until a rice-like texture is formed.

- These poppers can be stored in an airtight container in the fridge for up to 3 days or frozen for up to 3 months. Reheat in the oven at 350°F (180°C, or gas mark 5) until heated through.

Difficulty: **Easy**

Vegetarian | Low Carb | Gluten Free | Grain Free

Prep Time | 10 minutes

Cook Time | 20 minutes

Total Time | 30 minutes

Yield | 5 servings (20 poppers)

Calories Per Serving | 217

Total Carbs | 8 g

Net Carbs | 5 g

Protein | 11 g

Fat | 17 g

Ingredients:

2 cups (142 g) broccoli florets, finely diced (see notes)

½ cup (58 g) shredded cheddar cheese

1 cup (112 g) almond flour

1 garlic clove, minced

¼ teaspoon onion powder

¼ teaspoon chile flakes

½ teaspoon paprika

½ teaspoon salt

¼ teaspoon black pepper

2 large pasture-raised eggs, beaten

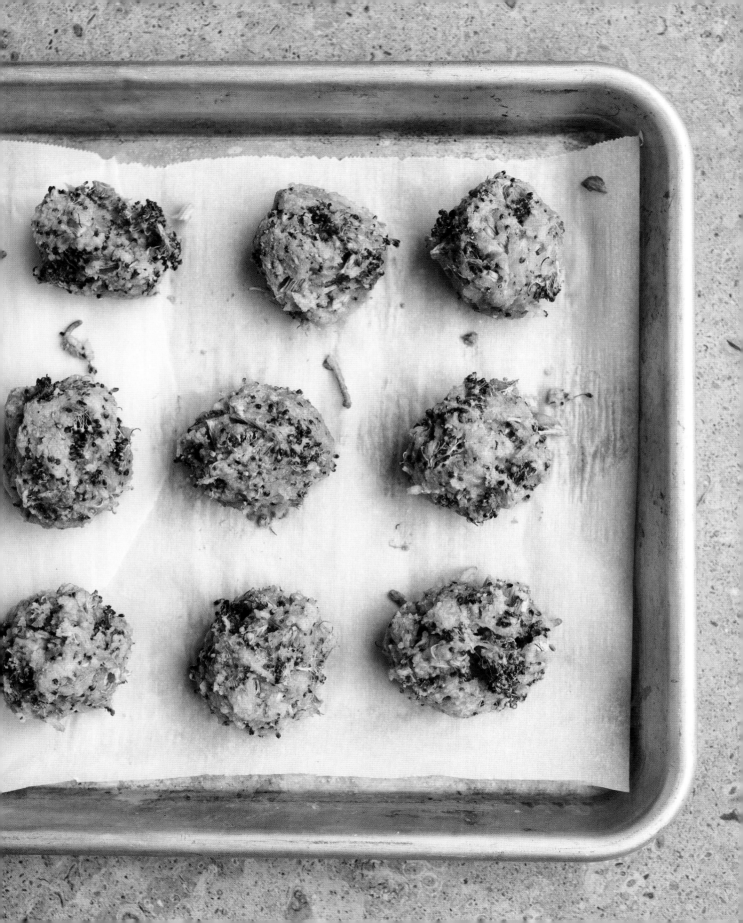

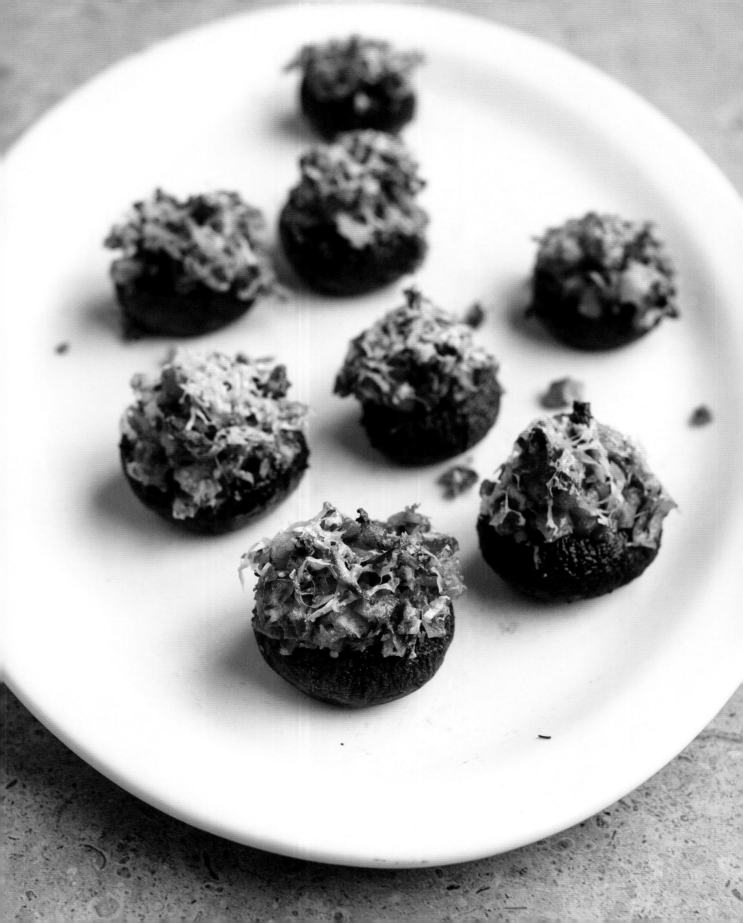

Stuffed Mushrooms

These nutty and fragrant stuffed mushrooms feature walnuts, chickpeas, and aromatic thyme for a protein-packed appetizer.

Instructions:

1. Preheat the oven to 400°F (200°C, or gas mark 6) and place the rack in the top third of the oven. Line a baking sheet with parchment paper.

2. Using a damp paper towel, wipe the mushrooms down, removing any dirt. Then, chop off the stems and reserve. Lay the mushroom caps evenly on the baking sheet, drizzle with a little olive oil, and set aside.

3. Dice the reserved mushroom stems. Add a little olive oil to a small saucepan over medium heat. Add the onion, mushroom stems, and garlic and cook until fragrant and soft, about 5 minutes. Add the walnuts and thyme and cook until toasted, about a minute. Remove from the heat and set aside.

4. In a small bowl, combine the chickpeas, half of the Parmesan cheese, parsley, salt, and pepper. Use a fork to mash the chickpeas and form a paste. Add the nut mixture to the chickpea mixture and stir well to combine.

5. Evenly spoon the filling into the mushroom caps and sprinkle the remaining Parmesan cheese on top.

6. Bake in the oven until the mushrooms are cooked through and the cheese has melted, about 15 minutes. Serve immediately while hot.

Notes

Please be aware that any ingredient additions, omissions, or substitutions will affect the nutritional information.

- Walnuts work best in this recipe, but you can also use pecans or any other nut of your choosing.
- Avoid washing the mushrooms as they will soak up too much liquid and will not bake well. Simply wipe them down with a damp paper towel.

Difficulty: **Easy**

Vegetarian | Low Carb | Gluten Free | Grain Free | Egg Free

Prep Time | 10 minutes

Cook Time | 15 minutes

Total Time | 25 minutes

Yield | 6 servings

Calories Per Serving | 119

Total Carbs | 6 g

Net Carbs | 4 g

Protein | 4 g

Fat | 9 g

Ingredients:

- 18 medium mushrooms
- 2 tablespoons (28 ml) olive oil
- ¼ small onion, finely diced
- 1 garlic clove, minced
- ¼ cup (30 g) chopped walnuts
- 1 tablespoon (4 g) dried thyme
- ½ cup (120 g) canned chickpeas, drained
- ¼ cup (25 g) grated Parmesan cheese
- 1 tablespoon (4 g) chopped fresh parsley
- ¼ teaspoon salt
- ¼ teaspoon black pepper

2

Post-Workout

High Protein, Higher Carbs, Lower Fats

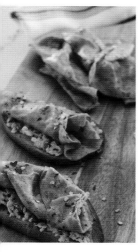

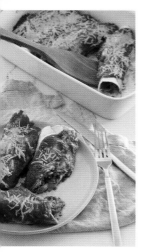

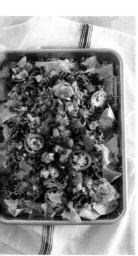

Post-workout nutrition is all about refilling the tank and giving your body what it needs to replenish and recover from your weights session at the gym. That's why we focus on high-quality animal-based proteins like beef, chicken, fish, and eggs in these recipes. These ingredients are packed full of essential amino acids to promote muscle growth and recovery.

Most of the recipes in this chapter also feature some healthy fats in moderation, like avocado, nuts, grass-fed butter, and olive oil because regardless of your fitness goals, as women we need dietary fats to maintain healthy hormone production. Essential fatty acids also help nutrient absorption so the body can shuttle all these important nutrients straight to where they need to go.

But the star of the post-workout plate really comes down to carbohydrates. An intense session of lifting weights will deplete your glycogen stores (remember the "fuel in the tank" analogy!). Refilling that empty tank after your workout is a surefire way to stoke that metabolism and get those muscles refueled.

Timing is also important when it comes to post-workout nutrition, and the recipes in this chapter are designed to be quick and easy to prepare, so you can refuel your body fast. Whether you're in the mood for a protein-packed smoothie or something a little more hearty, these recipes provide a variety of sweet and savory options that can be prepared ahead of time in bulk or made on the go when hunger strikes.

Apricot Breakfast Bake

Like a casserole but made with all your favorite porridge ingredients, this apricot breakfast bake is a comforting and hearty post-workout meal featuring succulent dried apricots, cinnamon, and crunchy walnuts.

Instructions:

1. Preheat the oven to 350°F (180°C, or gas mark 4) and place the rack placed in the middle of the oven. Line an 8 x 8-inch (20 x 20-cm) pan with parchment paper.

2. In a medium bowl, combine the oats, protein powder, coconut sugar, half of the walnuts (reserve the rest), baking powder, cinnamon, nutmeg, and salt. Mix well to combine.

3. In another bowl, beat the eggs and then whisk in the milk and vanilla extract until well combined. Add the wet ingredients to the dry ingredients and stir to combine. Add the butter and stir again until fully incorporated.

4. Evenly spread out the apricots and raisins over the bottom of the baking dish, reserving a few for the top. Pour in oatmeal mixture and spread evenly. Sprinkle with the remaining walnuts, raisins, and apricots.

5. Bake for 45 minutes to an hour until the walnuts on top are browned and the oats are set. Remove from the oven and let cool for 5 minutes before serving.

Notes

- Make sure to use rolled oats, not instant oats; otherwise, your breakfast bake will turn out mushy.
- When choosing a protein powder, use a high-quality, clean protein powder from grass-fed cows with no additives, fillers, gums, or anti-caking agents.

Difficulty: **Easy**

High Carb | Vegetarian | Gluten Free

Prep Time | 15 minutes

Cook Time | 1 hour

Total Time | 1 hour, 15 minutes

Yield | 6 servings

Calories Per Serving | 413

Total Carbs | 61 g

Net Carbs | 56 g

Protein | 20 g

Fat | 15 g

Ingredients:

2 cups (192 g) gluten-free rolled oats

2 scoops protein powder

⅔ cup (96 g) coconut sugar

½ cup (60 g) chopped walnuts, chopped

1 teaspoon baking powder

2 teaspoons ground cinnamon

¼ teaspoon ground nutmeg

½ teaspoon salt

2 large pasture-raised eggs

1⅔ cups (395 ml) full-fat cow's milk or nut milk of your choosing

1 teaspoon pure vanilla extract

1 tablespoon (14 g) unsalted grass-fed butter, melted

½ cup (85 g) dried apricots, chopped

¼ cup (35 g) raisins

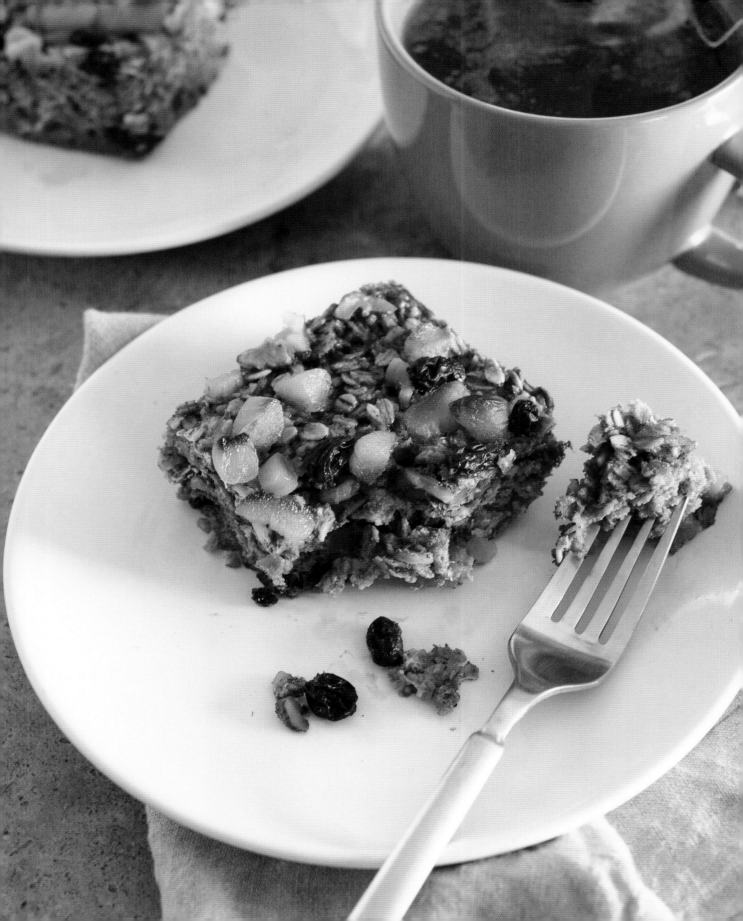

Banana Protein Pancakes

Who doesn't love pancakes for breakfast? This banana and oatmeal version is light, fluffy, and packed full of protein—a delicious and satisfying way refuel after an early morning workout.

Instructions:

1. Add all the ingredients to a blender and process until you have a smooth batter. If you prefer a thinner consistency, you can add more milk.

2. Heat a little olive oil or butter to a skillet pan over medium heat. Scoop a third of a cup (80 ml) of the batter onto the pan and cook for 2 to 3 minutes on each side or until golden brown with bubbles starting to form on the edges. Transfer the pancakes to serving plate.

3. Wipe the skillet down with a paper towel, add a little olive oil or butter again, and repeat with the remaining batter.

4. Serve with a drizzle of maple syrup, if desired.

Notes

Please be aware that any ingredient additions, omissions, or substitutions will affect the nutritional information.

- When choosing a protein powder, use a high-quality clean protein powder from grass-fed cows with no additives, fillers, gums, or anti-caking agents.

- For a nut-free option, use the full-fat cow's milk or a gluten-free, plant-based milk.

- You can also add toppings such as sliced bananas, berries, or nuts to make the pancakes even more delicious.

- You can make these pancakes in bulk ahead of time and store them with a piece of parchment paper separating each pancake in an airtight container for up to 5 days in the fridge or in the freezer. Simply warm them up on a parchment-lined baking sheet in the oven for 10 to 15 minutes on 300°F (150°C, or gas mark 2). Or if frozen, pop them in the toaster on a medium setting.

Difficulty: **Easy**

High Carb | High Protein | Gluten Free | Nut Free (optional)| Vegetarian

Prep Time | 10 minutes

Cook Time | 20 minutes

Total Time | 30 minutes

Yield | 3 servings (6 pancakes)

Calories Per Serving | 396

Total Carbs | 58 g

Net Carbs | 50 g

Protein | 29 g

Fat | 8 g

Ingredients:

2 large ripe bananas

2 large pasture-raised eggs

1½ cups (144 g) gluten-free rolled oats

2 scoops vanilla protein powder

2 teaspoons baking powder

½ teaspoon ground cinnamon

½ cup (120 ml) full-fat cow's milk or any nut milk of your choice (see notes)

1 teaspoon pure vanilla extract

1 tablespoon (15 ml) 100% pure maple syrup (optional)

Olive oil or grass-fed butter, for cooking

Cherry Chocolate Masa Bowl

This warm and comforting porridge recipe is perfect for a sweet post-workout breakfast. Made with masa harina, a finely ground corn flour, this porridge is high in carbohydrates, yet gluten free.

Instructions:

1. In a small mixing bowl, mix the masa harina with the water and almond milk. Let sit for at least an hour or overnight. This will ensure your porridge ends up with a creamy texture with no lumps.

2. In a medium saucepan, whisk together the masa harina mixture, collagen powder, honey, vanilla, and salt. Bring the mixture to a light boil over medium-high heat, stirring constantly to prevent lumps. Reduce the heat to low and simmer for 10 to 15 minutes, stirring occasionally, until the porridge has thickened and is creamy.

3. Once the porridge has thickened, slowly add the egg whites and whisk vigorously until fully combined and cooked through, about 2 to 3 minutes. Transfer to a serving bowl.

4. Add the raw egg yolk, cherries, and chocolate on top, drizzle with honey, and serve!

Notes

Please be aware that any ingredient additions, omissions, or substitutions will affect the nutritional information.

- For a nut-free option, use a gluten-free, plant-based milk or full-fat cow's milk.
- When choosing collagen powder, use a high-quality, clean collagen powder from grass-fed cows with no additives, fillers, gums, or anti-caking agents.
- For a vegetarian option, omit the collagen powder.
- Raw egg yolks are nutritious and perfectly safe to consume as long as you use high-quality pasteurized eggs and take care to store them safely.

Difficulty: **Easy**

High Carb | Vegetarian (optional) | Gluten Free | Nut Free (optional)	
Prep Time	1 hour, 5 minutes
Cook Time	20 minutes
Total Time	1 hour, 25 minutes
Yield	1 serving
Calories Per Serving	509
Total Carbs	55 g
Net Carbs	55 g
Protein	27 g
Fat	21 g

Ingredients:

- ¼ cup (29 g) masa harina
- ½ cup (120 ml) water
- ½ cup (120 ml) almond milk or other milk of choice (see notes)
- 1 scoop collagen powder (optional)
- 2 teaspoons raw honey, plus more to drizzle
- 1 teaspoon pure vanilla extract
- ¼ teaspoon salt
- 2 large pasture-raised eggs, yolks and whites separated
- ¼ cup (36 g) cherries, pitted
- 2 squares 70–80% dark chocolate

New York Deli Breakfast Burrito

Golden tender potatoes and pastrami in a burrito? Sold! This fusion breakfast might seem a little weird, but once you taste this hearty and flavorful New York Jewish deli–inspired breakfast burrito, you'll wonder where it's been all your life.

Instructions:

1. In a large skillet, heat a little olive oil over medium heat. Add the onion and garlic and cook until softened and fragrant, about 2 to 3 minutes.

2. Add the potatoes and cook until golden brown and tender, stirring occasionally, about 10 to 12 minutes.

3. Add the pastrami to the skillet and cook for another 2 to 3 minutes until heated through.

4. Crack the eggs into the skillet and scramble with the potato mixture. Season with dill, salt, and pepper.

5. Warm the tortillas on a separate skillet or in a warm oven for a few minutes. Spread a thin layer of mustard down the center of each tortilla.

6. Divide the egg and potato mixture between the tortillas and top each one with dill pickle rounds.

7. Roll up the tortilla to form a burrito and serve.

Difficulty: **Easy**

High Carb | High Protein | Nut Free | Dairy Free | Vegetarian (optional)

Prep Time | 10 minutes

Cook Time | 25 minutes

Total Time | 35 minutes

Yield | 2 servings

Calories Per Serving | 451

Total Carbs | 53 g

Net Carbs | 48 g

Protein | 26 g

Fat | 15 g

Ingredients:

Olive oil, for cooking

½ onion, chopped

1 garlic clove, minced

2 large potatoes, peeled and diced

3 ounces (85 g) pastrami, chopped (see notes)

3 large pasture-raised eggs

1 teaspoon dried dill

¼ teaspoon salt

¼ teaspoon black pepper

2 large flour tortillas

2 teaspoons Dijon mustard

1 dill pickle spear, thinly sliced into rounds

Notes

Please be aware that any ingredient additions, omissions, or substitutions will affect the nutritional information.

- For a vegetarian option, omit the pastrami and add sautéed mushrooms and bell peppers instead.
- You can make this burrito ahead of time, wrap it up tightly in parchment paper, and it should keep well in the fridge for 3 to 4 days.

StrongCurves

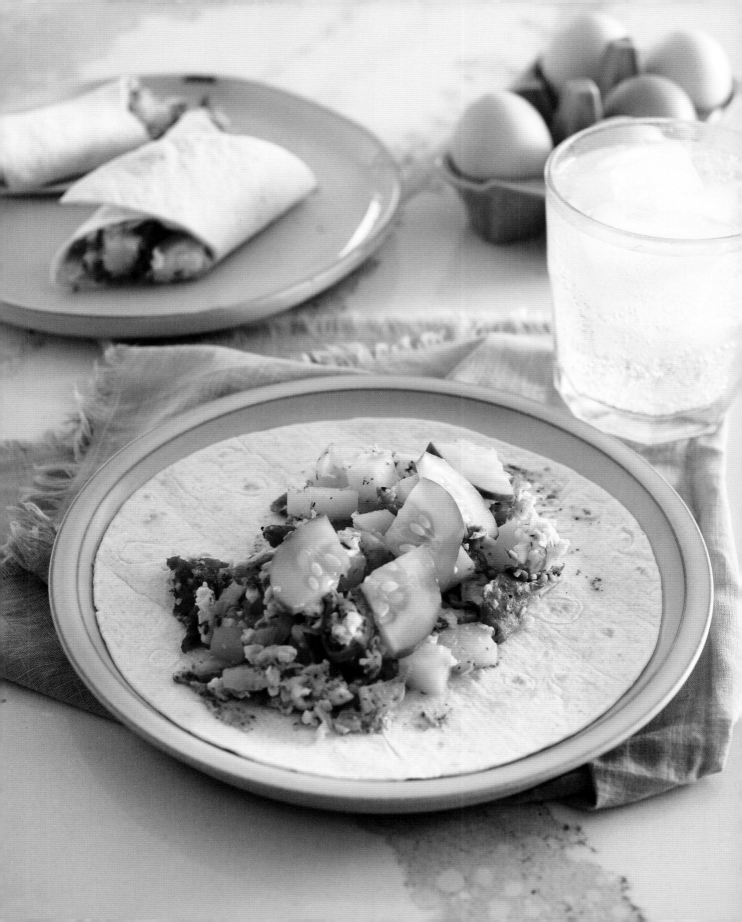

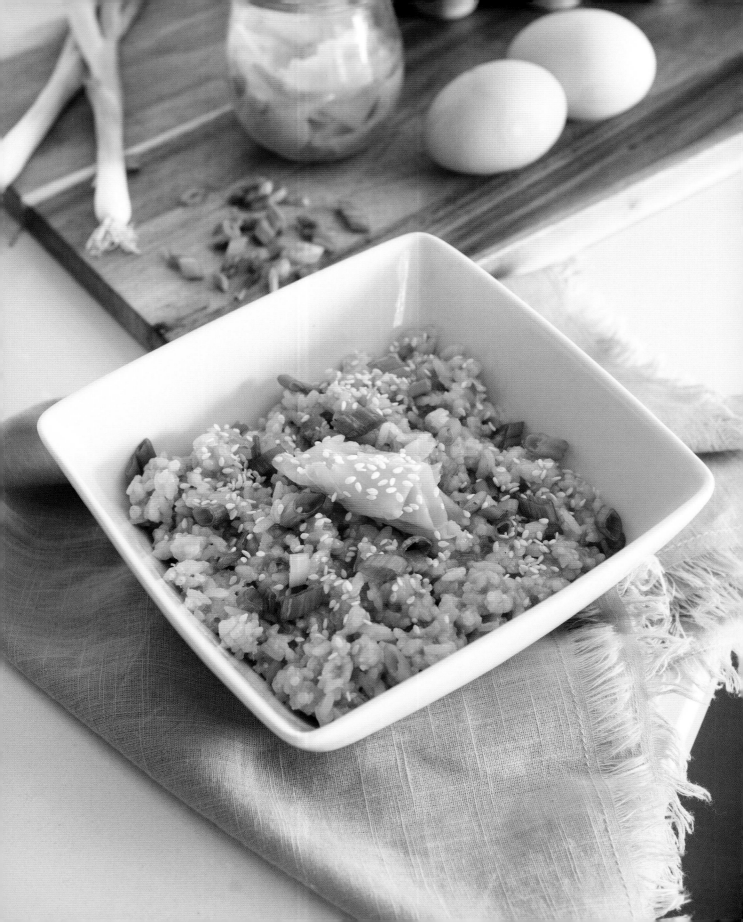

Japanese-Style Egg and Rice

A traditional Japanese breakfast dish, Tamago Kake Gohan is a simple but delicious rice bowl topped with a raw egg and seasonings. It's a popular way to start the day and provides a great source of protein and carbs to refuel after your workout.

Instructions:

1. Cook the rice according to package instructions using the chicken bone broth in place of water and place it in a serving bowl.

2. While the rice is piping hot, crack the eggs over the top, add the coconut aminos, and stir vigorously so that the eggs cook slightly. The rice should have a creamy consistency.

3. Garnish with green onion, sesame seeds, and pickled ginger and serve immediately.

Notes

- Make the Healing Bone Broth (page 166) ahead of time to use in this recipe. Alternatively, you can buy premade bone broth or stock, but make sure it's from pasture-raised high-quality chicken bones.
- Don't worry about using raw eggs in this recipe. As long as you use high-quality pasteurized eggs, it's perfectly safe to eat and the heat of the rice will gently cook the egg.

Difficulty: **Easy**

Prep Time | 5 minutes

Cook Time | 15 minutes

Total Time | 20 minutes

Yield | 1 serving

Calories Per Serving | 468

Total Carbs | 57 g

Net Carbs | 56 g

Protein | 26 g

Fat | 10 g

Ingredients:

1 cup (200 g) short-grain rice

1½ cups (355 ml) Healing Bone Broth (page 166) or store-bought chicken bone broth (see notes)

2 large pasture-raised eggs, raw

½ tablespoon coconut aminos or tamari

1 green onion, thinly sliced

½ teaspoon sesame seeds

1 tablespoon (15 g) pickled ginger

Savory Oatmeal with a Poached Egg

If you've never had savory oatmeal, you're truly missing out. Just like Goldilocks mused, the perfect bowl is not too sweet, but not too salty . . . it's just right. This recipe calls for comforting oats cooked in broth, topped with a runny egg and fried shallots for some extra crunch.

Instructions:

1. In a medium saucepan, bring the chicken bone broth to a boil. Add the rolled oats and stir to combine. Reduce the heat to low, cover, and simmer for 10 minutes, stirring occasionally until you reach your desired consistency. Season with salt and pepper. Transfer to a serving bowl.

2. While the oatmeal is cooking, poach the eggs. Bring a large pot of water to a boil and add the vinegar. Stir the water with a spatula to create a whirlpool and crack the eggs into the center of the pot. Let the eggs poach until the whites solidify but the yolk remains runny, about 3 to 4 minutes. Remove from the pot and set aside.

3. Heat a little coconut oil in a small skillet over medium heat. Add the shallot and garlic and cook for 2 to 3 minutes until fragrant. Remove from the heat and set aside.

4. Top the oatmeal with the poached eggs. Add the fried shallots and garlic on top. Sprinkle with chile flakes and drizzle with the coconut aminos.

5. Serve immediately and enjoy!

Notes

- Make the Healing Bone Broth (page 166) ahead of time to use in this recipe. Alternatively, you can buy premade bone broth or stock, but make sure it's from pasture-raised high-quality chicken bones.
- For a vegetarian option, substitute vegetable broth for the chicken bone broth.
- You can cook your eggs to your preference whether fried, boiled, or poached, but make sure the yolks are still runny as this works best with this recipe.

Difficulty: **Easy**

High Carb | Vegetarian (optional)| Gluten Free | Dairy Free | Nut Free

Prep Time | 5 minutes

Cook Time | 15 minutes

Total Time | 20 minutes

Yield | 1 serving

Calories Per Serving | 387

Total Carbs | 48 g

Net Carbs | 44 g

Protein | 29 g

Fat | 12 g

Ingredients:

1 cup (235 ml) Healing Bone Broth (page 166) or store-bought chicken bone broth or vegetable broth (see notes)

½ cup (48 g) gluten-free rolled oats

¼ teaspoon salt

¼ teaspoon black pepper

2 large pasture-raised eggs

Dash of white vinegar, for poaching

Coconut oil, for cooking

½ shallot, diced

1 garlic clove, minced

¼ teaspoon chile flakes

½ tablespoon coconut aminos or tamari

Strong*Curves*

Sweet Potato and Turkey Quinoa Bowl

With roasted sweet potato, fluffy quinoa, and a variety of fresh vegetables, this filling bowl is a great source of protein and packed with whole carbs.

Instructions:

1. Preheat the oven to 400°F (200°C, or gas mark 6) and place the rack in the middle of the oven. Line a baking sheet with parchment paper.

2. Place the sweet potato on a baking sheet and drizzle with a little olive oil. Season with salt and pepper and toss to coat. Roast for 25 to 30 minutes or until tender and lightly browned.

3. While the sweet potato is roasting, prepare the quinoa. Add the quinoa and chicken bone broth to a medium saucepan and bring to a boil. Reduce the heat to low, cover, and simmer for 15 to 20 minutes or until the quinoa is tender and the water is absorbed.

4. In a large skillet over medium heat, add a little olive oil. When the skillet is hot, add the ground turkey and season with cumin, paprika, salt, and pepper. Use your cooking utensil to break up the ground turkey in the pan and cook until it's browned and cooked through, about 6 to 8 minutes.

5. In a large bowl, combine the quinoa, roasted sweet potato, turkey, cabbage, cherry tomatoes, salad greens, pepitas, lemon juice, and cilantro. Toss well to combine.

6. Divide the mixture among four bowls and serve immediately.

Notes

Please be aware that any ingredient additions, omissions, or substitutions will affect the nutritional information.

- Make the Healing Bone Broth (page 166) ahead of time to use in this recipe or use a high-quality store-bought bone version
- Ground beef, chicken, or pork also works well in this recipe.

Difficulty: Easy

High Protein | High Carb | Gluten Free | Dairy Free | Nut Free | Egg Free

Prep Time | 10 minutes

Cook Time | 35 minutes

Total Time | 45 minutes

Yield | 4 servings

Calories Per Serving | 499

Total Carbs | 44 g

Net Carbs | 37 g

Protein | 40 g

Fat | 19 g

Ingredients:

1 large sweet potato, cubed

Olive oil, for cooking

½ teaspoon salt, divided

¼ teaspoon black pepper, divided

2 cups (346 g) quinoa, rinsed

4 cups (946 ml) Healing Bone Broth (page 166) or store-bought chicken bone broth (see notes) or water

1 pound (455 g) ground turkey

½ tablespoon ground cumin

½ tablespoon smoked paprika

¼ cup (18 g) red cabbage, thinly sliced

1 cup (150 g) cherry tomatoes, halved

2 cups (110 g) mixed salad greens

2 tablespoons (18 g) pepitas

½ lemon, juiced

¼ cup (4 g) fresh cilantro, chopped

Shakshuka (Eggs Poached in Tomato Sauce)

This classic Middle Eastern tomato-based dish is just the right amount of spicy, rich, and satisfying. High in muscle-building protein and paired with a serving of Bone Broth Rice (page 110) or Mushroom Pearl Couscous (page 108), it's a perfect way to refuel after a heavy gym session.

Instructions:

1. Heat the butter in a large skillet over medium heat. Add the onion and garlic and sauté for 2 to 5 minutes until soft and translucent.

2. Add the cherry tomatoes and parsley and cook until the tomatoes start to release their liquid, about 5 minutes. Add the paprika, cumin, chile flakes, salt, and pepper, stirring well to combine. Use the back of a wooden spoon to gently squash the tomatoes until they burst their skin.

3. Add the broth and tomato paste to the pan and stir to combine. Bring to a boil and then lower the heat to simmer until the sauce reduces and thickens, about 5 to 10 minutes. Add more broth if necessary to keep the sauce from drying out.

4. Make 6 holes in the sauce and crack an egg in each one. Season each egg with a little salt and pepper and cover the pan with a lid. Cook for 3 to 5 minutes or until the egg whites are cooked through and yolks still runny.

5. Remove from the heat and serve immediately (the eggs will continue to cook in the hot pan, so be careful not to overcook).

Notes

- For a vegetarian option, substitute vegetable broth for the chicken bone broth.
- For strict low-carb and keto-friendly, simply enjoy the dish as is without the rice or couscous.

Difficulty: **Moderate**

Vegetarian (optional) | High Protein | Gluten Free | Nut Free | Keto Friendly (optional)

Prep Time | 10 minutes

Cook Time | 20 minutes

Total Time | 30 minutes

Yield | 2 servings

Calories Per Serving | 346

Total Carbs | 12 g

Net Carbs | 9 g

Protein | 24 g

Fat | 20 g

Ingredients:

1 tablespoon (14 g) grass-fed butter or ghee

½ small yellow onion, finely diced

2 garlic cloves, minced

1½ cups (225 g) cherry tomatoes, halved

3 tablespoons (12 g) chopped fresh parsley

2 teaspoons smoked paprika

½ teaspoon ground cumin

½ teaspoon chile flakes

1 teaspoon pink Himalayan rock salt

¼ teaspoon black pepper

1 cup (235 ml) Healing Bone Broth (page 166) or store-bought chicken bone broth or vegetable broth (see notes)

1 tablespoon (16 g) tomato paste

6 large pasture-raised eggs

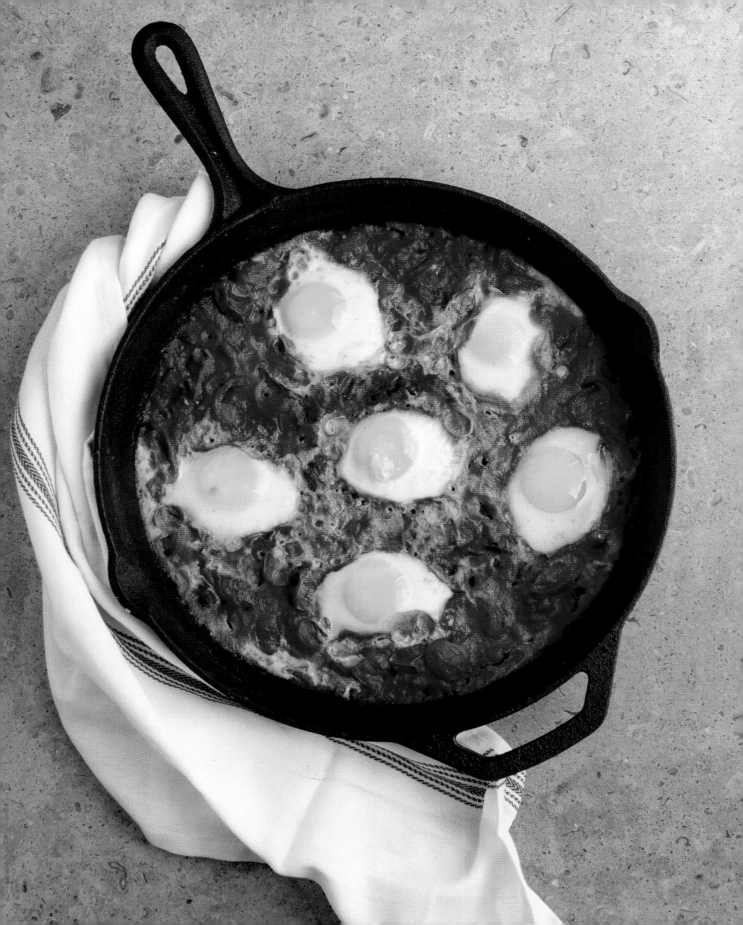

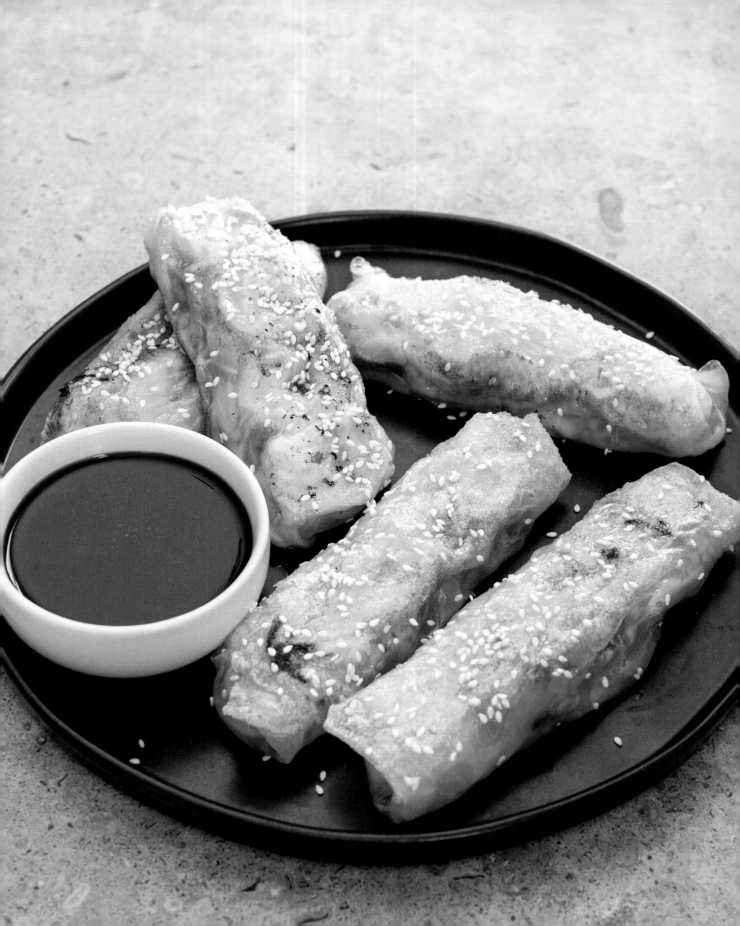

Crispy Shrimp Rice Paper Rolls

These healthier homemade Asian-style crispy rolls are filled with succulent shrimp and flavorful vegetables. They're packed full of protein and gluten-free carbs.

Instructions:

1. Add a little sesame oil to a skillet over medium-high heat, about a teaspoon. Add the green onion, garlic, and ginger and sauté until fragrant, about 1 minute.

2. Add the bean sprouts, cabbage, carrot, mushrooms, salt, and pepper to the pan and cook until tender but still crisp, about 2 to 3 minutes. Do not overcook or the rice paper rolls will be soggy. Remove from the heat, transfer to a large bowl, and set aside to cool.

3. In the same skillet, add a little more sesame oil and add the shrimp. Cook for 1 to 2 minutes each side until cooked through. Remove from the heat and set aside.

4. To assemble the rolls, dip 2 rice paper rolls in cold water for a few seconds so they're pliable but not too sticky. Lay them on top of each other on a damp paper towel so that they don't stick to your work surface while you assemble the rolls.

5. Place 4 shrimp in the center of the rice paper wrapper and then top with a heaped tablespoon (15 ml) of the veggie mixture. Fold the bottom of the wrapper up over the filling and then fold in the sides and roll tightly, like a burrito. Repeat with the remaining wrappers and filling.

6. Add a little coconut oil to a large skillet over medium-high heat. When the pan is hot, add the rice paper rolls 2 at a time, frying on each side for 2 to 3 minutes or until golden and crispy. Repeat for the remaining rolls and add a little more coconut oil if needed.

7. To make the dipping sauce, whisk together the coconut aminos, honey, and rice vinegar in a small mixing bowl.

8. Serve the Crispy Shrimp Rice Paper Rolls hot, sprinkle them with sesame seeds, and serve with the dipping sauce on the side.

Difficulty: **Moderate**

High Protein | High Carb | Pescatarian | Gluten Free | Nut Free | Egg Free

Prep Time | 15 minutes

Cook Time | 15 minutes

Total Time | 30 minutes

Yield | 5 rolls

Calories Per Roll | 215

Total Carbs | 31 g

Net Carbs | 30 g

Protein | 22 g

Fat | 3 g

Ingredients:

FOR THE ROLLS:

Sesame oil, for cooking

1 green onion, finely chopped

1 garlic clove, minced

1 tablespoon (8 g) grated fresh ginger

½ cup (52 g) bean sprouts

½ cup (35 g) shredded cabbage

½ cup (55 g) shredded carrot

½ cup (70 g) shitake mushrooms, sliced

¼ teaspoon salt

¼ teaspoon black pepper

20 large shrimp, peeled and deveined

10 rice paper wrappers

Coconut oil, for frying

1 teaspoon sesame seeds

FOR THE DIPPING SAUCE:

2 tablespoons (28 ml) coconut aminos or tamari

1 tablespoon (20 g) raw honey

1 tablespoon (15 ml) rice vinegar

BLT Pasta Salad

Juicy tomatoes, crisp lettuce, creamy avocado, and smoky bacon bits make this carb-rich dish a family favorite. With fresh and simple ingredients, you can whip it up in under 20 minutes for a satisfying post-workout lunch.

Instructions:

1. Cook the fusilli pasta according to package instructions. Drain and set aside to cool.

2. Bring a pot of water to a rolling boil. Add the eggs and cook for 8 minutes or until hard boiled. Remove from the heat and run under cold water. Set aside. Once cooled, peel and half the eggs.

3. While the eggs and pasta are cooking, prepare the bacon. In a skillet over medium heat, cook the turkey bacon until crispy, about 6 to 8 minutes. Remove from heat and set aside.

4. In a large mixing bowl, combine the cherry tomatoes, romaine lettuce, avocado, and red onion. Toss to combine. Add the cooked pasta and turkey bacon. Season with dried oregano, salt, and pepper and mix well to combine.

5. Chill the pasta salad in the refrigerator for at least 30 minutes before serving. When ready to serve, divide the pasta salad between 4 bowls and top each bowl with 2 eggs.

Notes

Please be aware that any ingredient additions, omissions, or substitutions will affect the nutritional information.

- For a gluten-free option, substitute gluten-free pasta for the regular pasta.
- You can use pork bacon in place of turkey bacon; however, choose a leaner cut such as center-cut bacon.

Difficulty: **Easy**

High Carb | Low Fat | Vegetarian | Nut Free | Gluten Free (optional)

Prep Time | 10 minutes

Cook Time | 15 minutes

Chill Time | 30 minutes

Total Time | 55 minutes

Yield | 4 servings

Calories Per Serving | 460

Total Carbs | 49 g

Net Carbs | 44 g

Protein | 26 g

Fat | 17 g

Ingredients:

8 ounces (225 g) fusilli pasta (see notes)

8 large pasture-raised eggs

6 slices turkey bacon, chopped

2 cups (300 g) cherry tomatoes, halved

4 cups (188 g) romaine lettuce, chopped

½ avocado, cubed

1 tablespoon (10 g) thinly sliced red onion

1 teaspoon dried oregano

Salt and black pepper, to taste

Tuna and Mayo Topped Baked Potato

A hot and fluffy baked potato topped with a creamy tuna salad is a simple yet deliciously satisfying lunch filled with healthy carbohydrates and protein.

Instructions:

1. Preheat the oven to 350°F (180°C, or gas mark 4) and place the rack in the middle of the oven. Place the potato on a baking sheet and bake in the oven for 1 hour or until tender.

2. While the potato is baking, prepare the tuna salad. In a medium bowl, combine the tuna, mayonnaise, sweet corn, lemon juice, and parsley. Season with salt and pepper to taste and stir until well combined.

3. Once the potato is cooked, remove it from the oven and let cool for a few minutes. Cut a slit down the center of the potato and gently push the sides in to make a pocket for the filling.

4. Spoon the tuna salad into the potato pocket. Serve hot and enjoy!

Notes

When buying store-bought mayonnaise, look for high-quality brands that use olive oil or avocado oil rather than vegetable or seed oils and avoid preservatives and additives. Or use your favorite recipe to make your own homemade mayonnaise!

Difficulty: **Easy**

High Carb | High Protein | Pescatarian | Grain Free | Gluten Free | Nut Free

Prep Time | 10 minutes

Cook Time | 1 hour

Total Time | 1h, 10 minutes

Yield | 1 serving

Calories Per Serving | 404

Total Carbs | 45 g

Net Carbs | 40 g

Protein | 37 g

Fat | 8 g

Ingredients:

1 large baking potato, washed and skin pierced with a fork

1 can (5 ounces, or 140 g) tuna in water, drained

1 tablespoon (14 g) olive oil mayonnaise

¼ can (15 ounces, or 425 g) sweet corn, drained

½ lemon, juiced

½ tablespoon chopped fresh parsley

Salt and black pepper, to taste

Taco Nachos with Salsa

A Mexican staple, these cheesy loaded beef nachos are just the right amount of spicy and crunchy, topped with zesty salsa. Easy to whip together in under 20 minutes, this is the perfect recipe for those days when you come back from the gym in need of sustenance fast!

Instructions:

1. Preheat the oven to 350°F (180°C, or gas mark 4) and place the rack in the top third of the oven.

2. In a large skillet, heat a little olive oil over medium-high heat. Add the ground beef and cook until browned, breaking up the meat with a wooden spoon as it cooks. Drain any excess fat.

3. Add the chili powder, cumin, garlic powder, paprika, oregano, salt, and pepper, stirring to combine. Stir in the refried black beans. Cook for 5 to 7 minutes until the mixture has thickened slightly.

4. Arrange the tortilla chips in a single layer on a baking sheet. Spoon the beef mixture over the chips, making sure to distribute it evenly. Sprinkle the cheddar cheese over the top.

5. Bake the nachos in the oven for 10 to 12 minutes or until the cheese is melted and bubbly.

6. While the nachos are cooking, prepare the salsa. In a medium bowl, add the salsa ingredients and stir to combine.

7. When the nachos are done, remove them from the oven and let cool for a few minutes. Spoon the salsa over the top of the nachos, making sure to distribute it evenly. Serve while hot and enjoy!

Difficulty: **Easy**

High Protein | High Carb | Gluten Free | Egg Free | Nut Free

Prep Time | 10 minutes

Cook Time | 12 minutes

Total Time | 22 minutes

Yield | 6 servings

Calories Per Serving | 442

Total Carbs | 37 g

Net Carbs | 34 g

Protein | 25 g

Fat | 23 g

Ingredients:

FOR THE TACO NACHOS:

Olive oil, for cooking

1 pound (455 g) lean ground beef

½ teaspoon chili powder

½ teaspoon ground cumin

½ teaspoon garlic powder

1 teaspoon paprika

1 teaspoon oregano

½ teaspoon salt

¼ teaspoon black pepper

1 can (16 ounces, or 455 g) refried black beans

½ cup (58 g) shredded cheddar cheese

1 bag (size varies) gluten-free tortilla chips

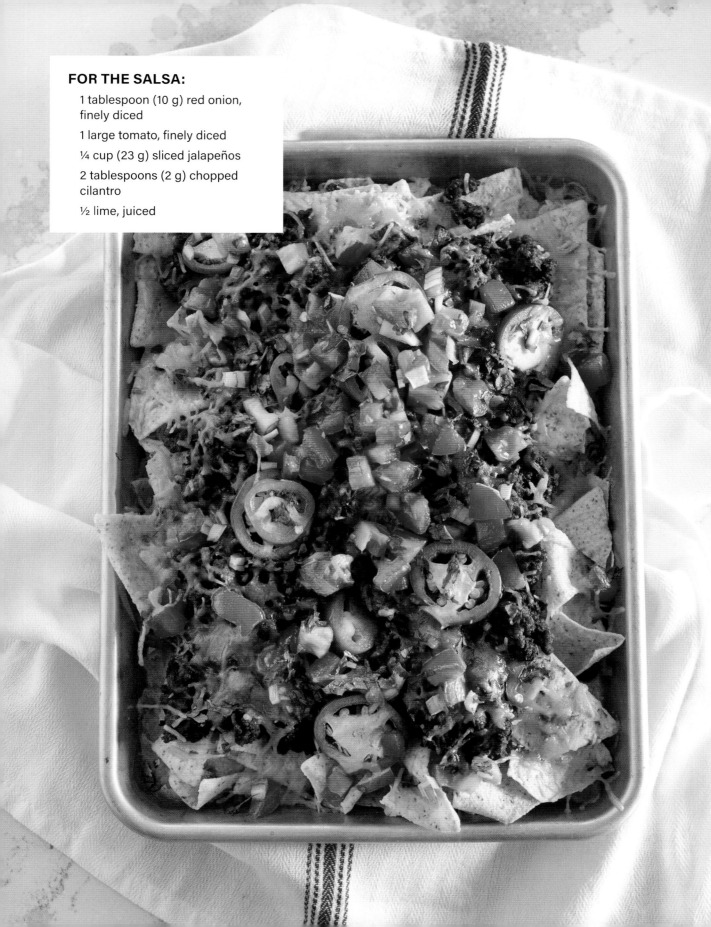

FOR THE SALSA:

1 tablespoon (10 g) red onion, finely diced

1 large tomato, finely diced

¼ cup (23 g) sliced jalapeños

2 tablespoons (2 g) chopped cilantro

½ lime, juiced

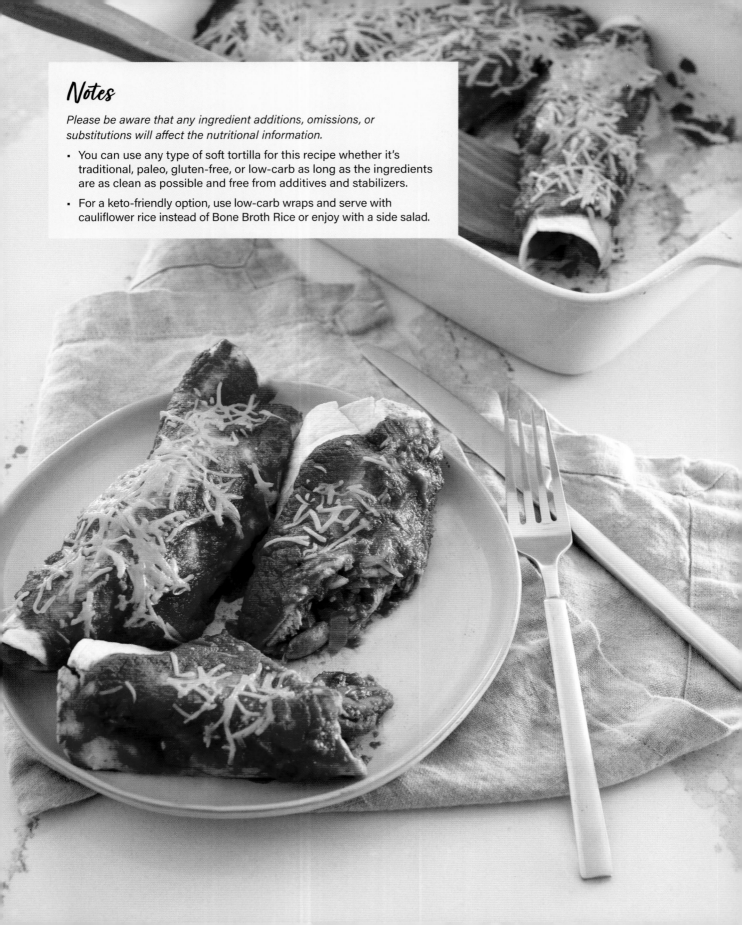

Notes

Please be aware that any ingredient additions, omissions, or substitutions will affect the nutritional information.

- You can use any type of soft tortilla for this recipe whether it's traditional, paleo, gluten-free, or low-carb as long as the ingredients are as clean as possible and free from additives and stabilizers.

- For a keto-friendly option, use low-carb wraps and serve with cauliflower rice instead of Bone Broth Rice or enjoy with a side salad.

Chicken Enchiladas

A Mexican staple that's as great for midweek dinners and entertaining guests as it is as a post-workout meal. Serve with Bone Broth Rice (page 110).

Instructions:

1. Preheat the oven to 350°F (180°C, or gas mark 4) and place the rack in the middle of the oven. Grease a large baking sheet and set aside.

2. Add all the spices, salt, and pepper to a small bowl and stir until combined.

3. To make the sauce, add the tomato purée and half of the spice mixture to a small saucepan and gently simmer over medium heat. Let it reduce for 10 minutes or so until slightly thickened. Set to one side until you're ready to assemble the enchiladas.

4. Start making the enchilada filling while the sauce is simmering. Heat the olive oil in a large skillet over medium heat and add the onion and garlic. Sauté for a few minutes until soft and translucent. Add the chicken and the rest of the spice mixture to the skillet and cook for 5 minutes, stirring regularly until browned. Add the mushrooms and bell pepper and cook for another 5 minutes until the bell pepper have softened and the mushrooms release their liquid. Remove pan from the heat and set aside.

5. To assemble the enchiladas, arrange the chicken filling, sauce, tortilla wraps, and cheddar cheese in a line formation. Place a tortilla on a plate and spoon a few tablespoons (45 to 60 ml) of the sauce onto the tortilla, spreading it evenly but leaving a ¾ inch (2 cm) gap along the edge. Add some of the filling in a line down the center of the wrap and top with a small sprinkle of cheese. Roll one side of the wrap over the other and place the enchilada carefully in the baking sheet, seam-side down. Repeat with the rest of the tortillas, packing them closely together.

6. Pour the remaining sauce evenly over the top of the tortillas and sprinkle the remaining cheese on top. Garnish with cilantro and bake for a 20 minutes until cheese is golden.

Difficulty: **Moderate**

High Carb | High Protein | Nut Free | Keto Friendly (optional)

Prep Time | 10 minutes

Cook Time | 45 minutes

Total Time | 55 minutes

Yield | 6 servings

Calories Per Serving | 423

Total Carbs | 42 g

Net Carbs | 39 g

Protein | 35 g

Fat | 12 g

Ingredients:

1 teaspoon ground cumin

½ teaspoon mild chili powder

1 teaspoon dried oregano

½ teaspoon paprika

Salt and black pepper, to taste

1½ cups (375 g) tomato purée

1 teaspoon olive oil

1 medium onion, finely diced

1 garlic clove, minced

4 chicken breasts (6 ounces, or 170 g each), cut into thin strips ½ inch (1.3 cm) in thickness

1 cup (70 g) button mushrooms, sliced

1 red bell pepper, sliced into strips

6 soft tortilla wraps

½ cup (58 g) shredded cheddar cheese

1 tablespoon (1 g) chopped cilantro (optional)

Red Thai Curry with Shrimp

This traditional Thai recipe calls for succulent tiger shrimp in a creamy red curry sauce with fragrant lemon grass, cilantro, and basil. It's super easy to make using simple whole food ingredients and can be whipped up in under 30 minutes with a side of jasmine rice for a quick post-workout dinner.

Instructions:

1. Prepare the jasmine rice according to package instructions.

2. Add half of the coconut milk to a large wok or skillet over medium heat and bring to a simmer. Add the red curry paste and stir continuously for 3 to 5 minutes until the coconut milk reduces and the paste thickens. Then, add the remaining coconut milk and bring to a simmer, stirring to combine.

3. Stir in the lemon grass, coconut aminos, coconut sugar, and garlic. Add the shrimp, bell pepper, snow peas, baby corn, bamboo shoots, and bean sprouts and cook for another 3 to 5 minutes until the vegetables have slightly softened and shrimp have cooked through.

4. Remove from the heat, add the lime juice and basil leaves, and stir through.

5. Divide the rice between 4 serving bowls. Ladle the curry on top, garnish with cilantro, and serve.

Notes

Please be aware that any ingredient additions, omissions, or substitutions will affect the nutritional information.

- You can substitute any meat or fish of your choice for the shrimp.
- For a low-carb option, substitute cauliflower rice or zucchini noodles for the rice or simply enjoy the dish on its own!
- Leftovers can be stored in an airtight container in the refrigerator for up to 3 days.

Difficulty: **Easy**

High Protein | High Carb | Pescatarian | Gluten Free | Dairy Free | Egg Free | Nut Free

Prep Time | 10 minutes

Cook Time | 15 minutes

Total Time | 25 minutes

Yield | 4 servings

Calories Per Serving | 506

Total Carbs | 56 g

Net Carbs | 54 g

Protein | 31 g

Fat | 19 g

Ingredients:

1 cup (200 g) jasmine rice

1 can (13½ ounces, or 380 g) coconut milk

2 tablespoons (30 g) Thai red curry paste

1 stalk lemongrass, bruised

1 tablespoon (15 ml) coconut aminos or tamari

1 tablespoon (9 g) coconut sugar

2 garlic cloves, minced

20 tiger or king shrimp, peeled and deveined

½ red bell pepper, sliced

½ cup (32 g) snow peas

½ cup (110 g) baby corn

½ cup (66 g) bamboo shoots, drained

½ cup (52 g) bean sprouts, drained

1 tablespoon (15 ml) lime juice

¼ cup (6 g) Thai or regular basil leaves, chopped

Cilantro, chopped to garnish

Strong*Curves*

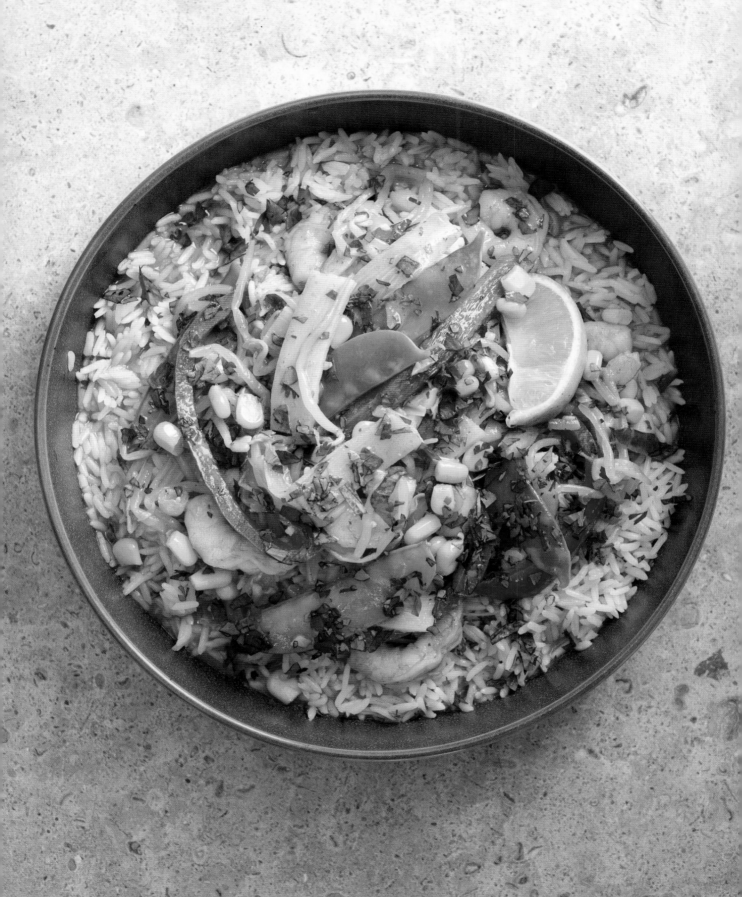

Salmon Sushi Bake

A deconstructed take on a Japanese staple, this salmon sushi bake has all the delicious elements of a sushi roll without the need for the fiddly assembly.

Instructions:

1. Preheat the oven to 400°F (200°C, or gas mark 6) and place the rack in the middle of the oven.

2. Cook the rice according to package instructions and set aside. Once cooled slightly, transfer to a mixing bowl. Add half the rice vinegar, stir well to combine, and then add the remaining vinegar and stir again to combine.

3. While the rice is cooking, season the salmon with salt, pepper, garlic powder, and paprika and place on a baking sheet skin-side down. Bake in the oven for 10 to 12 minutes until cooked through but slightly pink in the center. Remove from the oven, allow to cool down, transfer to a separate mixing bowl, and then flake it using a fork. Discard the skin. Add the cream cheese, mayonnaise, and sriracha to the salmon. Mix well and set aside.

4. Transfer your rice to a casserole dish and spread it evenly across the bottom, pressing it down with a spatula to create a flat layer that completely covers the bottom of the dish. Sprinkle the crumbled seaweed sheets over the top of the rice to create a layer of seaweed that completely covers the rice. Use as many seaweed sheets as needed.

5. Add the salmon mixture on top and evenly spread it over the seaweed sheet layer. Turn the oven down to 375°F (190°C, or gas mark 5) and bake for 10 minutes until the salmon is slightly golden and crunchy. Remove from the oven and let cool for a few minutes.

6. Top the casserole with a drizzle of sriracha and mayonnaise, sesame seeds, and green onion. Serve and enjoy!

Difficulty: **Easy**

High Protein | High Carb | Pescatarian | Gluten Free | Nut Free

Prep Time | 10 minutes

Cook Time | 22 minutes

Total Time | 32 minutes

Yield | 5 servings

Calories Per Serving | 461

Total Carbs | 31 g

Net Carbs | 31 g

Protein | 30 g

Fat | 23 g

Ingredients:

3 cups (390 g) white rice

¼ cup (60 ml) rice vinegar

3 large salmon filets, skin on

¼ teaspoon salt

¼ teaspoon black pepper

¼ teaspoon garlic powder

¼ teaspoon paprika

¼ cup (60 g) full-fat cream cheese

¼ cup (60 g) olive oil mayonnaise, plus more to garnish

2 tablespoons (28 ml) sriracha, plus more to garnish

4–5 seaweed sheets, crumbled

1 tablespoon (8 g) black sesame seeds

2 tablespoons (12 g) chopped green onion

Chili Con Carne

A Mexican favorite that incorporates tender ground beef and flavorful spices in a rich tomato sauce, this dish can be made in bulk to last many meals throughout the week.

Instructions:

1. Cook the rice according to package instructions.

2. Heat a little olive oil in a large pot over medium heat. Add the garlic and onions and sauté until soft, about 2 minutes. Add the bell pepper and cook until softened, about 5 minutes.

3. Add the ground beef to the pot and cook until browned, breaking it up with a spatula into small pieces as it cooks, about 8 minutes. Drain any excess fat from the pot if needed and return it to the heat.

4. Add the cumin, oregano, paprika, cayenne pepper, salt, and black pepper and stir to combine. Continue to cook for 2 to 3 minutes.

5. Add the diced tomatoes, tomato paste, kidney beans, and bone broth and stir well to combine. Reduce the heat to medium-low. Simmer for 1 to 1½ hours until the chili has reduced and thickened.

6. Divide the rice into serving bowls, top with a portion of the chili, and garnish with cilantro.

Notes

Please be aware that any ingredient additions, omissions, or substitutions will affect the nutritional information.

- You can use any lean ground meat in place of beef, such as turkey, chicken, or pork.

- For a vegetarian option, you can omit the meat and add extra beans and vegetables.

- Make the Healing Bone Broth (page 166) ahead of time to use in this recipe. Alternatively, you can buy premade bone broth or stock, but make sure it's from pasture-raised high-quality chicken bones.

- Leftovers can be stored in the refrigerator for up to 3 days.

Difficulty: **Easy**

High Protein | High Carb | Gluten Free | Dairy Free | Nut Free

Prep Time | 10 minutes

Cook Time | 1 hour, 30 minutes

Total Time | 1 hour, 40 minutes

Yield | 4 servings

Calories Per Serving | 460

Total Carbs | 37 g

Net Carbs | 32 g

Protein | 39 g

Fat | 17 g

Ingredients:

2 cups (380 g) white rice

Olive oil, for cooking

2 garlic cloves, minced

2 yellow onions, chopped

1 green bell pepper, diced

2 pounds (900 g) lean ground beef

1 tablespoon (7 g) ground cumin

1 tablespoon (3 g) dried oregano

2 teaspoons smoked paprika

½ teaspoon cayenne pepper

1½ teaspoons salt

¼ teaspoon black pepper

2 cans (14 ounces, or 390 g each) diced tomatoes

2 tablespoons (32 g) tomato paste

1 cup (256 g) canned kidney beans, drained and rinsed

½ cup (120 ml) bone broth (see notes)

1 tablespoon chopped cilantro, to garnish

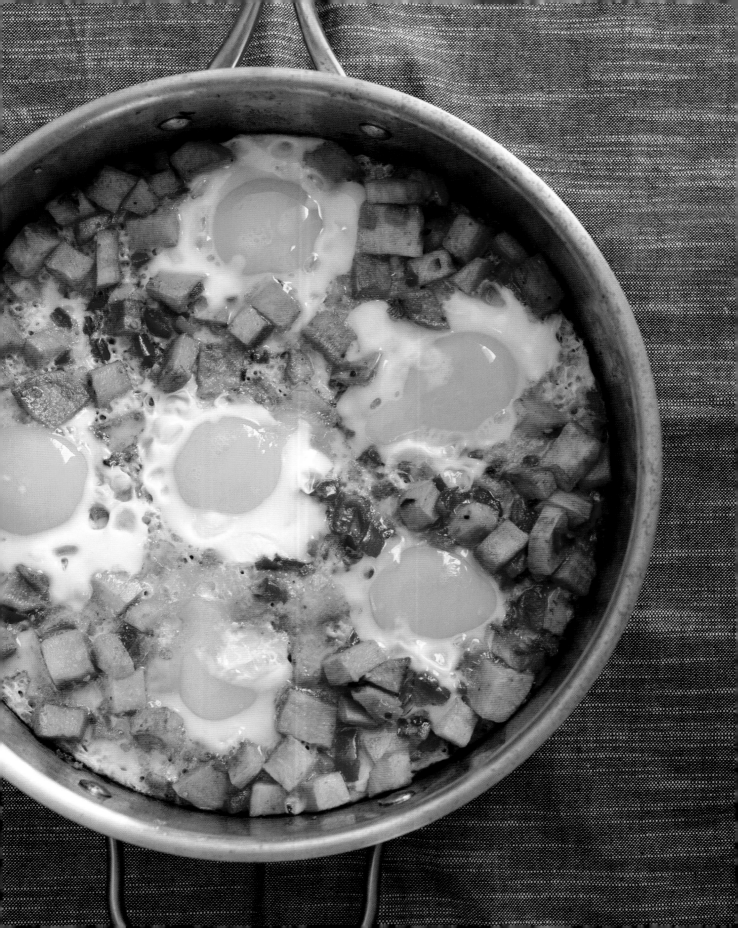

One Pan Moroccan Potato Hash

With fragrant spices, panfried sweet potato, and gooey eggs, this Moroccan-style hash can be enjoyed at any time of the day! The beauty of cooking it all in one pan means you can whip up a delicious post-workout meal in no time at all . . . and spend less time washing dishes after!

Instructions:

1. Preheat a large skillet over medium-high heat. Add a little olive oil and swirl to coat the pan.

2. Add the red onion, bell pepper, and garlic to the skillet. Sauté until slightly soft, about 2 to 3 minutes.

3. Push the vegetables to the side of the skillet and add the sweet potatoes, paprika, cumin, turmeric, chili powder, cinnamon, salt, and pepper and cook until golden brown and crispy, stirring regularly to ensure even cooking, about 8 minutes. Make sure to occasionally stir the vegetables so that they don't burn at the side of the pan.

4. Once the potatoes are cooked through, start to mix the vegetables in with the potatoes and cook for another 2 minutes.

5. Using a spatula, make 6 wells in the mixture and crack an egg in each one. Cover the pan and lower the heat to medium-low and cook until the whites are cooked through but yolks are still runny, about 5 minutes.

6. Remove the skillet from the heat and let it rest for a few minutes. Use a spatula to divide the hash mixture and eggs into two servings.

7. Serve hot and enjoy!

Notes

Please be aware that any ingredient additions, omissions, or substitutions will affect the nutritional information.

For a low-carb version, substitute an equivalent amount of cauliflower florets for the sweet potatoes.

Difficulty: **Easy**

High Protein | High Carb | Vegetarian | Gluten Free | Grain Free | Nut Free

Prep Time | 10 minutes

Cook Time | 20 minutes

Total Time | 30 minutes

Yield | 2 servings

Calories Per Serving | 410

Total Carbs | 34 g

Net Carbs | 29 g

Protein | 22 g

Fat | 25 g

Ingredients:

Olive oil, for cooking

¼ red onion, finely diced

1 red bell pepper, diced

2 garlic cloves, minced

2 large sweet potatoes, peeled and cubed into ½ inch (1.3 cm) pieces

½ teaspoon paprika

½ teaspoon ground cumin

½ teaspoon ground turmeric

½ teaspoon chili powder

Pinch of ground cinnamon

½ teaspoon salt

¼ teaspoon black pepper

6 large pasture-raised eggs

Beef and Rice Stuffed Peppers

Cheesy rice and tender beef in a rich tomato sauce make these stuffed peppers a no-brainer when you're hungry and ready to refuel after a weights session.

Instructions:

1. Preheat the oven to 375°F (190°C, or gas mark 5) and place the rack in the middle of the oven.

2. Cook the rice according to package instructions and set aside.

3. Place the bell peppers upside down in a large casserole dish, drizzle with olive oil, season with a little salt and pepper, and roast in the oven for 15 to 20 minutes until softened and slightly browned. Remove from the heat and set aside.

4. Heat a little olive oil in a large skillet over medium-high heat. Add the onion and garlic to the skillet and cook for 2 to 3 minutes until softened. Add the ground beef and cook until browned, breaking it up into small pieces with a wooden spoon. Stir in the oregano, chili powder, cumin, paprika, salt, and pepper. Cook for an additional 2 to 3 minutes until well combined. Pour in the tomato purée and bring to a boil.

5. Reduce the heat to medium-low and cook for another 2 to 3 minutes until the sauce has thickened. Add the rice and half of the cheddar cheese and stir to combine. Remove from the heat and set aside.

6. Turn the bell peppers over in the baking dish so the open side is facing up. Stuff each pepper by spooning the beef and rice mixture into the center cavity and sprinkle with the remaining cheese. When all the peppers are stuffed, return the baking dish to the oven and bake for 10 to 15 minutes until the peppers are tender and the cheese is bubbly and golden.

7. Serve hot!

Difficulty: **Easy**

High Protein | High Carb | Gluten Free | Nut Free | Egg Free

Prep Time | 10 minutes

Cook Time | 35 minutes

Total Time | 45 minutes

Yield | 4 servings

Calories Per Serving | 545

Total Carbs | 43 g

Net Carbs | 40 g

Protein | 40 g

Fat | 23 g

Ingredients:

2 cups (380 g) white rice

4 large red bell peppers, tops cut off, seeds and core removed

Olive oil, for cooking

1¼ teaspoons salt, divided

¼ teaspoon black pepper, divided

1 medium yellow onion, finely chopped

2 garlic cloves, minced

1 pound (455 g) lean ground beef

½ teaspoon dried oregano

½ teaspoon chili powder

½ teaspoon ground cumin

1 teaspoon paprika

1 cup (250 g) tomato purée

1½ cups (173 g) shredded cheddar cheese

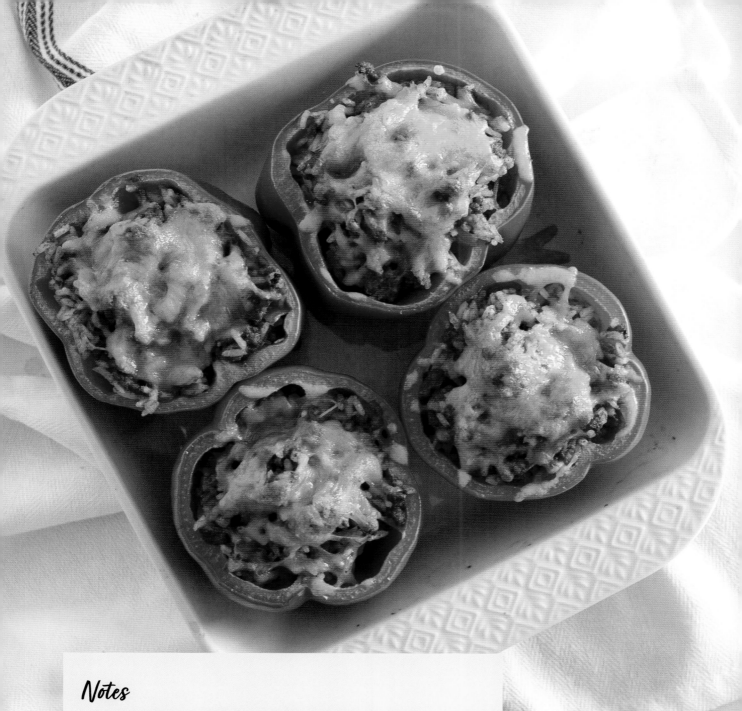

Notes

Please be aware that any ingredient additions, omissions, or substitutions will affect the nutritional information.

- Leftovers can be stored in the refrigerator for up to 3 days. To reheat, simply bake in the oven until warmed through.

- Any lean ground meat can be used such as chicken, turkey, lamb, or pork.

- Make sure to use equal sized peppers with flat bottoms so that they cook evenly and stand upright in the casserole dish.

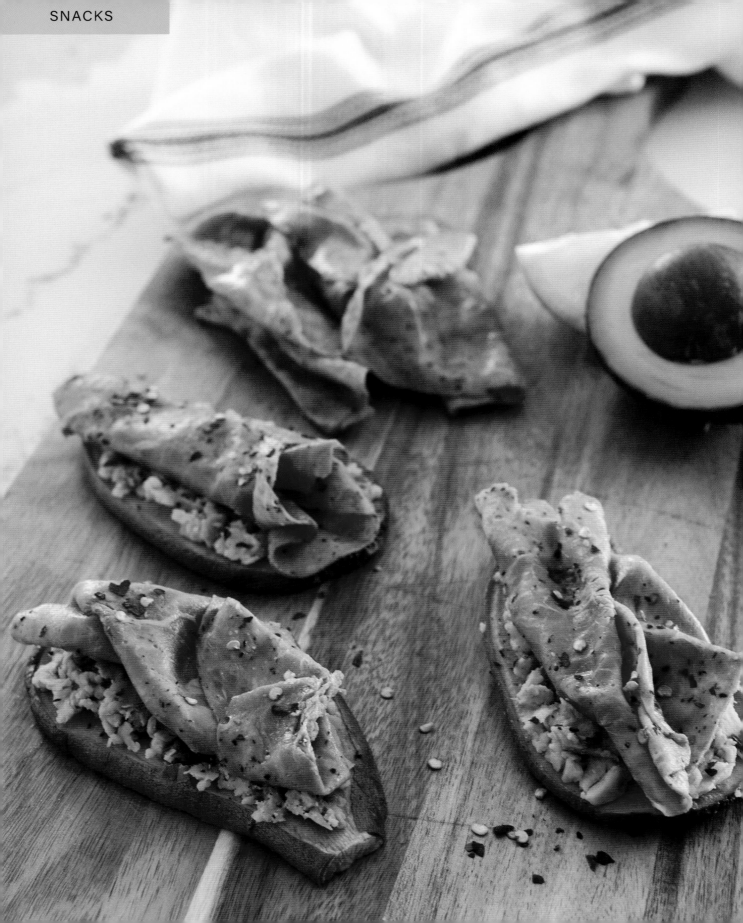

Sweet Potato Avocado Boats

A twist on everyone's favorite avocado toast, this recipe uses golden sweet potatoes and succulent pastrami for a satisfying gluten-free post-workout snack.

Instructions:

1. Preheat the oven to 400°F (200°C, or gas mark 6) and place the rack in the top third of the oven.

2. Place the sweet potato on a baking sheet, brush the top with olive oil, and bake for 20 to 25 minutes or until tender and golden. Remove from the oven and let cool for a few minutes.

3. In a small mixing bowl, add the avocado and lemon juice and mix well to combine. Season with salt and pepper to taste.

4. Spread the avocado mixture evenly over the sweet potato slices and top each one with a slice of pastrami.

5. Serve immediately, garnished with chile flakes if desired.

Notes

Please be aware that any ingredient additions, omissions, or substitutions will affect the nutritional information.

You can use any protein in place of the pastrami, such a turkey slices, shredded chicken, or tuna.

Difficulty: **Easy**

High Protein | High Carb | Gluten Free | Grain Free | Egg Free | Nut Free | Dairy Free

Prep Time | 10 minutes

Cook Time | 25 minutes

Total Time | 35 minutes

Yield | 2 servings (6 boats)

Calories Per Serving | 262

Total Carbs | 25 g

Net Carbs | 20 g

Protein | 18 g

Fat | 11 g

Ingredients:

1 large sweet potato, sliced lengthwise into ½-inch (1.3 cm) thick slices (about 6 pieces)

Olive oil, for baking

½ ripe avocado, mashed

¼ lemon, juiced

Salt and black pepper, to taste

6 slices deli pastrami

¼ teaspoon chile flakes (optional)

Rice Cakes 3 Ways

Difficulty: **Easy**

High Carb | Gluten Free | Egg Free |

An easy post-workout snack that satisfies all your refueling needs, rice cakes are versatile and can be enjoyed with a variety of toppings, both savory and sweet.

Instructions:

1. Stack or spread each rice cake with the toppings listed, serve immediately, and enjoy.

OPTION 1: ALMOND BUTTER AND BANANA

Prep Time | 5 minutes

Total Time | 5 minutes

Yield | 1 serving

Calories Per Serving | 198

Total Carbs | 33 g

Net Carbs | 30 g

Protein | 5 g

Fat | 9 g

Ingredients:

1 large rice cake

1 tablespoon (16 g) almond butter

½ medium banana, sliced

1 teaspoon raw honey, to drizzle

OPTION 2: COTTAGE CHEESE AND AVOCADO

Yield | 1 serving

Calories Per Serving | 112

Total Carbs | 16 g

Net Carbs | 13 g

Protein | 6 g

Fat | 6 g

Ingredients:

1 large rice cake

2 tablespoons (28 g) high-protein cottage cheese

¼ avocado, sliced

Pinch of chile flakes

OPTION 3: HUMMUS, TURKEY, AND CHEESE

Yield | 1 serving

Calories Per Serving | 164

Total Carbs | 14 g

Net Carbs | 13 g

Protein | 12 g

Fat | 12 g

Ingredients:

1 large rice cake

1 tablespoon (15 g) hummus

1 slice turkey

1 slice cheddar cheese

StrongCurves

No-Bake Protein Bar

The ultimate grab-and-go post-workout snack, these healthy homemade protein bars are loaded with real food goodness. Make them ahead of time and pop one in a zip top bag to enjoy after your weights session. I promise you'll never go back to the processed version you get at the store!

Instructions:

1. Line an 8 x 8-inch (20 x 20-cm) baking dish with parchment paper.

2. In a large mixing bowl, add the protein powder and rolled oats and stir to combine.

3. In a small saucepan, add the almond butter and honey over low heat and mix well until smooth and melted.

4. Add the wet ingredients to the bowl of dry ingredients and stir until fully incorporated. If needed, add the almond milk a little at a time until a thick batter consistency is achieved. If your batter is crumbly, add more liquid.

5. Add the dark chocolate chips and mix everything together until well combined.

6. Pour the mixture into the dish and press down firmly to make an even layer.

7. Place in the refrigerator and let it set for at least 1 hour or until firm.

8. When ready to serve, remove from the fridge and slice into 8 even bars.

Difficulty: **Easy**

High Protein | High Carb | Gluten Free | Egg Free |

Prep Time | 10 minutes

Chill | 1 hour

Total Time | 1 hour, 10 minutes

Yield | 8 servings

Calories Per Serving | 224

Total Carbs | 26 g

Net Carbs | 23 g

Protein | 11 g

Fat | 9 g

Ingredients:

3 scoops vanilla protein powder

1 cup (96 g) gluten-free rolled oats

⅓ cup (87 g) almond butter or any nut/seed butter of your choosing

⅓ cup (115 g) raw honey

⅓ cup (80 ml) almond milk

¼ cup (60 g) unsweetened dark chocolate chips (optional)

Notes

Please be aware that any ingredient additions, omissions, or substitutions will affect the nutritional information.

- Store bars in an airtight container in the fridge for up to one week. You can use any nut milk of your choice or full-fat cow's milk.

- When choosing a protein powder, use a high-quality, clean protein powder from grass-fed cows with no additives, fillers, gums, or anti-caking agents.

Cinnamon Apple with Nut Butter

A delicious and filling snack is perfect for those looking for a high-protein AND high carb-option. These cinnamon apple slices with nut butter are easy to make and made with simple whole food ingredients. This recipe is great for pre- or post-workout fueling or for a healthy snack in between meals.

Instructions:

1. Arrange the apple slices on a plate.

2. In a small bowl, mix the peanut butter, protein powder, honey, and cinnamon until well combined.

3. Spread the peanut butter mixture onto the apple slices, dividing it evenly among them.

4. Serve immediately or store in an airtight container in the refrigerator for up to 24 hours.

Notes

Please be aware that any ingredient additions, omissions, or substitutions will affect the nutritional information.

- You can use any nut butter of your choosing, such as almond or cashew.
- For a nut-free option, substitute sunflower seed butter for the nut butter.
- When choosing a protein powder, use a high-quality, clean protein powder from grass-fed cows with no additives, fillers, gums, or anti-caking agents.

Difficulty: **Easy**

High Protein | High Carb | Gluten Free | Grain Free | Egg Free | Nut Free (optional)	
Prep Time | 10 minutes	
Total Time | 10 minutes	
Yield | 1 serving	
Calories Per Serving | 375	
Total Carbs | 49 g	
Net Carbs | 41 g	
Protein | 24 g	
Fat | 11 g	

Ingredients:

1 medium apple, sliced and core removed

1 tablespoon (16 g) natural peanut butter (see notes)

1 scoop vanilla protein powder

2 teaspoons raw honey

½ teaspoon ground cinnamon

Pesto Deviled Eggs

Hard boiled eggs with a fragrant pesto dip made with basil, crunchy pine nuts, and olive oil makes this recipe a filling high-protein snack after your workout.

Instructions:

1. Make the pesto ahead of time. Add the pine nuts to a food processor and pulse a few times until small, coarse pieces form. Do not overprocess! Add the remaining ingredients and pulse until the desired consistency is achieved. You may need to scrape down the sides a few times to ensure that the mixture is evenly processed. Pesto can be stored in a mason jar in the fridge for up to a week.

2. To make the deviled eggs, place the eggs in a large pot and fill with cold water so that the eggs are completely immersed with at least an inch (2.5 cm) of water above them. Bring the water to a full rolling boil and then switch the heat off, leaving the pot in place on the stove top. Cover with a lid and let sit for 10 to 12 minutes. Drain the hot water, leaving the eggs in the pot, and run cold water over the eggs to stop them from overcooking.

3. While the eggs are cooking, add ¼ cup (65 g) of pesto, mayonnaise, salt, and pepper into a small mixing bowl and stir to combine.

4. Peel the eggs under cold running water. Slice in half lengthwise and gently squeeze to remove the yolks into the mixing bowl with the pesto filling.

5. Mash the yolks into the filling with a fork and stir until well combined. Use a teaspoon to scoop the filling into the hollow egg whites and sprinkle with paprika.

6. Serve immediately or chill in the fridge for later.

Notes

Please be aware that any ingredient additions, omissions, or substitutions will affect the nutritional information.

For a dairy-free option, omit the Parmesan cheese.

Difficulty: **Easy**

High Protein | Gluten Free | Grain Free | Vegetarian | Dairy Free (optional)

Prep Time | 10 minutes

Cook Time | 12 minutes

Total Time | 22 minutes

Yield | 2 servings (12 deviled eggs)

Calories Per Serving | 363

Total Carbs | 3 g

Net Carbs | 2 g

Protein | 26 g

Fat | 6 g

Ingredients:

FOR THE DEVILED EGGS:

6 large pasture-raised eggs

2 tablespoons (28 g) olive oil mayonnaise

¼ teaspoon salt

¼ teaspoon black pepper

¼ teaspoon smoked paprika

FOR THE BASIL AND PINE NUT PESTO:

⅓ cup (45 g) pine nuts

⅓ cup (80 ml) olive oil

1 garlic clove

2 cups (48 g) fresh basil leaves

¼ teaspoon salt

¼ teaspoon black pepper

⅓ cup (33 g) grated Parmesan cheese (optional)

Herbed Latkes

Golden and crispy shredded potato cakes are more often enjoyed during the Jewish festival of Hanukkah, but they're delicious at any time of year, especially post-workout for a carb-rich side dish to any main meal.

Instructions:

1. As soon as the potatoes are grated, add them to a large bowl of cold water for 2 minutes. Drain in a colander and squeeze the excess liquid out using a cheesecloth.

2. Add the strained potato back into a large, dry mixing bowl along with the onion and stir to combine.

3. Stir in the matzo meal, eggs, potato starch, parsley, chives, salt, and pepper until well-combined.

4. Add a little avocado oil to a large skillet on medium-high heat. Scoop ¼ cup (60 ml) of the mixture at a time into your hands and form it into a tightly packed round patty. Drop a latke into the oil very gently. (The oil should sizzle, not smoke. Lower the heat a touch if it does.) Gently press the latke down with a spatula, making sure they keep their shape.

5. Cook the latke for 2 to 3 minutes per side until golden brown. Drain on a paper towel-lined rack. Repeat for the remaining mixture. You can fry up to 4 latkes at a time once you have the oil at the right temperature.

Notes

- Latkes can be stored in the fridge in an airtight container for up to a week.
- To reheat, place on a baking sheet and heat in an oven at 375°F (190°C, or gas mark 5) for about 10 minutes until heated through.

Difficulty: **Moderate**

High Carb | Grain Free | Gluten Free | Vegetarian | Dairy Free | Nut Free

Prep Time | 10 minutes

Cook Time | 25 minutes

Total Time | 35 minutes

Yield | 4 servings

Calories Per Serving | 249

Total Carbs | 49 g

Net Carbs | 45 g

Protein | 8 g

Fat | 3 g

Ingredients:

2½ pounds (1.1 kg) medium yellow potatoes, peeled and grated

1 large onion, grated

¾ cup (90 g) matzo meal or gluten-free breadcrumbs

2 large pasture-raised eggs, beaten

1 tablespoon (12 g) potato starch

1 tablespoon (4 g) chopped fresh parsley

½ tablespoon chopped chives

1¼ teaspoons salt

½ teaspoon black pepper

Avocado oil, for frying

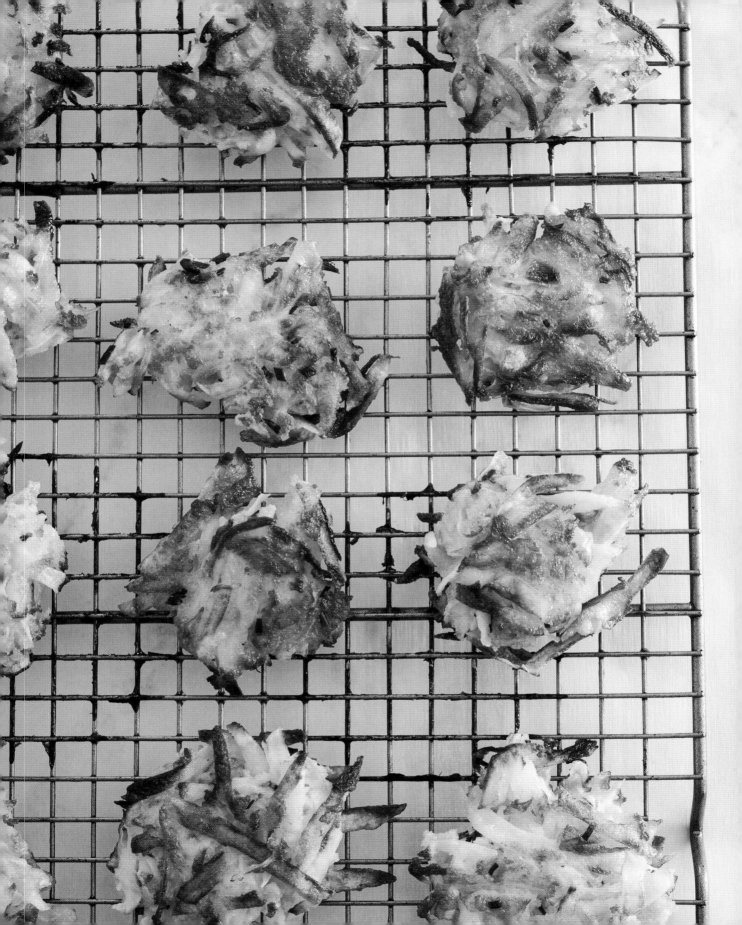

Mushroom Pearl Couscous

This carb-rich side dish is a staple in any Israeli home. You may not be familiar with pearl couscous, which isn't as well-known as it's finer and smaller cousin, Moroccan couscous. Pearl couscous is basically tiny fluffy balls of pasta. When combined with nourishing bone broth, mushrooms, and spinach, it makes for a delicious post-workout side that accompanies any main dish perfectly.

Instructions:

1. Add a little olive oil to a large skillet on medium heat. Add the onion and garlic and sauté until soft and translucent, about 3 minutes. Add the mushrooms and sauté until they release their liquid, about 5 minutes. Add the spinach, salt, and pepper and stir to combine. Cook until spinach is wilted, about 3 minutes. Remove from the heat and set aside.

2. Add a little olive oil to a medium saucepan over medium-high heat. When the oil is hot, add the couscous and stir to combine. Cook until the couscous is toasted and golden but not burnt, about 2 minutes.

3. Add the chicken bone broth, bring to a rolling boil, and then lower the heat to a simmer and cover. Cook until the liquid has evaporated, stirring occasionally, about 10 minutes.

4. Remove from the heat and add the mushroom mixture to the couscous. Stir to combine. Serve and enjoy!

Notes

Make the Healing Bone Broth (page 166) ahead of time to use in this recipe. Alternatively, you can buy premade bone broth or stock, but make sure it's from pasture-raised high-quality chicken bones.

Difficulty: **Easy**

High Carb | Dairy Free | Nut Free | Egg Free

Prep Time | 5 minutes

Cook Time | 25 minutes

Total Time | 30 minutes

Yield | 2 servings

Calories Per Serving | 245

Total Carbs | 32 g

Net Carbs | 28 g

Protein | 18 g

Fat | 6 g

Ingredients:

Olive oil, for cooking

1 small onion, sliced

2 garlic cloves, minced

1 cup (70 g) mushrooms, sliced

6 cups (180 g) spinach

½ teaspoon sea salt

¼ teaspoon black pepper

1 cup (171 g) Israeli pearl couscous

2 cups (475 ml) Healing Bone Broth (page 166) or store-bought chicken bone broth (see notes)

StrongCurves

Sweet Potato Fries

Lightly salted, oven baked, chunky sweet potato fries are a healthier homemade version of the fast food favorite. Dipped in in your favorite sauce, they're great carb-rich post-workout side for any main dish.

Instructions:

1. Preheat the oven to 425°F (220°C, or gas mark 7) and place the rack in the top third of the oven. Line a baking sheet with parchment paper.

2. Add the sweet potato fries to a large mixing bowl, drizzle with olive oil, and massage with your hands until evenly coated. Add the salt, pepper, paprika, and garlic powder and mix well to combine.

3. Spread the fries out onto the baking sheet, spacing them evenly and making sure they do not touch each other; otherwise, they will come out soggy.

4. Bake for 25 to 30 minutes, flipping them half way through with a spatula and turning the baking sheet in the oven to ensure even cooking.

Notes

- Make sure the fries are all cut the same size to avoid them cooking unevenly.
- Cooking time may need to be adjusted depending on if your oven runs hot or cool. Keep a close eye during the last 10 minutes of cooking.

Difficulty: **Easy**

High Carb | Gluten Free | Grain Free | Vegetarian | Dairy Free | Nut Free | Egg Free

Prep Time | 5 minutes

Cook Time | 30 minutes

Total Time | 35 minutes

Yield | 2 servings

Calories Per Serving | 228

Total Carbs | 38 g

Net Carbs | 31 g

Protein | 4 g

Fat | 8 g

Ingredients:

1 medium sweet potato, washed and sliced into ¼-inch (6 mm) strips

1 teaspoon olive oil

⅛ teaspoon salt

¼ teaspoon black pepper

1 teaspoon smoked paprika

¼ teaspoon garlic powder

Bone Broth Rice

Supercharged rice made with nourishing chicken bone broth is rich in essential amino acids, collagen, and carbs, making this a perfect post-workout side with any main dish.

Instructions:

1. Add the rice, chicken bone broth, and butter or ghee to a saucepan and bring to a boil over medium-high heat.

2. Cover, reduce the heat to medium-low, and simmer for 12 minutes or until the water has fully absorbed. Remove from the heat and allow to sit for 10 minutes.

3. Fluff the rice up with a fork, season with salt and pepper, and serve with your main dish.

Notes

Please be aware that any ingredient additions, omissions, or substitutions will affect the nutritional information.

- Use any rice of your choosing, but be aware that cooking times may differ.
- Make the Healing Bone Broth (page 166) ahead of time to use in this recipe. Alternatively, you can buy premade bone broth or stock, but make sure it's from pasture-raised high-quality chicken bones.
- For a dairy-free option, omit the grass-fed butter or ghee.

Difficulty: **Easy**

High Carb | Gluten Free | Dairy Free (optional) | Nut Free | Egg Free

Prep Time | 5 minutes

Cook Time | 22 minutes

Total Time | 27 minutes

Yield | 2 servings

Calories Per Serving | 401

Total Carbs | 75 g

Net Carbs | 74 g

Protein | 10 g

Fat | 4 g

Ingredients:

1 cup (200 g) jasmine rice, rinsed

1¼ cups (295 ml) Healing Bone Broth (page 166) or store-bought chicken bone broth (see notes)

2 teaspoons unsalted grass-fed butter or ghee (optional)

Salt and pepper, to taste

Peanut Butter Banana Smoothie

Deliciously creamy and thick, this post-workout protein-packed smoothie tastes just like a diner milkshake but is so much healthier. Made with real food ingredients including quinoa (yes, quinoa in a smoothie!), it's a great option if you're short on time, but still want a balanced and filling meal replacement. Simply blend and go!

Instructions:

1. Prepare the quinoa ahead of time according to package instructions and set aside to cool.

2. In a blender, add the banana, cooled quinoa, peanut butter, protein powder, honey, unsweetened almond milk, vanilla extract, cinnamon, salt, and ice cubes.

3. Blend the ingredients on high speed for 1 to 2 minutes or until the mixture is smooth and creamy. Add more almond milk if you prefer a looser consistency.

4. Pour the smoothie into a glass and enjoy immediately.

Notes

- This recipe calls for cooked quinoa for a smoothie texture. You can use uncooked quinoa to save even more time, as long as your blender is powerful enough. However, the texture will be grittier but still delicious!

- When choosing a protein powder, use a high-quality, clean protein powder from grass-fed cows with no additives, fillers, gums, or anti-caking agents.

- For a vegetarian option, omit the protein powder.

Difficulty: **Easy**

High Protein | High Carb | Vegetarian (optional) | Grain Free | Gluten Free | Dairy Free | Egg Free

Prep Time | 5 minutes

Total Time | 5 minutes

Yield | 1 serving

Calories Per Serving | 470

Total Carbs | 48 g

Net Carbs | 38 g

Protein | 29 g

Fat | 16 g

Ingredients:

¼ cup (46 g) cooked quinoa

1 frozen banana

1 tablespoon (16 g) natural peanut butter or any nut butter of your choice

1 scoop vanilla protein powder (optional)

1 teaspoon raw honey

1 cup (235 ml) unsweetened almond milk or any nondairy milk of your choice

½ teaspoon pure vanilla extract

¼ teaspoon ground cinnamon

Pinch of salt

4–5 ice cubes

Green Goddess Smoothie

This fruity and fresh drink gets its name from all the gorgeous green fruits and vegetables packed full of antioxidants, fiber, and healthy fats that goes into it. If you struggle to get your daily veggies in, this Green Goddess Smoothie is an easy and delicious solution that can be enjoyed post-workout or really any time of the day.

Instructions:

1. Add all the ingredients into a blender and process on high speed for 1 to 2 minutes or until the mixture is smooth and creamy. Add a little water if you prefer a looser consistency.

2. Pour the smoothie into a glass and enjoy immediately.

Notes

Please be aware that any ingredient additions, omissions, or substitutions will affect the nutritional information.

- This recipe is so versatile, you can substitute any of the fruit and vegetables to your preference such as apples, grapes, celery, or kale—just as long as they're green!

- I recommend using a 1:1 ratio of fruit to vegetables to ensure your smoothie has the right amount of sweetness. If you prefer it sweeter, simply add a little more fruit or add your favorite natural sweetener such a raw honey or 100% pure maple syrup.

- When choosing a protein powder, use a high-quality, clean protein powder from grass-fed cows with no additives, fillers, gums, or anti-caking agents.

- For a vegetarian option, omit the protein powder.

- For a dairy-free option, substitute an equivalent amount of coconut yogurt or coconut milk for the Greek yogurt.

Difficulty: **Easy**

High Protein | High Carb | Vegetarian (optional) | Grain Free | Gluten Free | Egg Free | Nut Free | Dairy Free (optional)

Prep Time | 5 minutes

Total Time | 5 minutes

Yield | 1 serving

Calories Per Serving | 452

Total Carbs | 57 g

Net Carbs | 45 g

Protein | 34 g

Fat | 12 g

Ingredients:

¼ ripe avocado

1 cup (43 g) baby spinach, washed

1 small ripe pear, peeled and core removed

1 kiwi fruit, peeled and halved

½ small cucumber, peeled and chopped

1 scoop vanilla protein powder (optional)

½ cup (115 g) full-fat Greek yogurt (see notes)

4–6 ice cubes

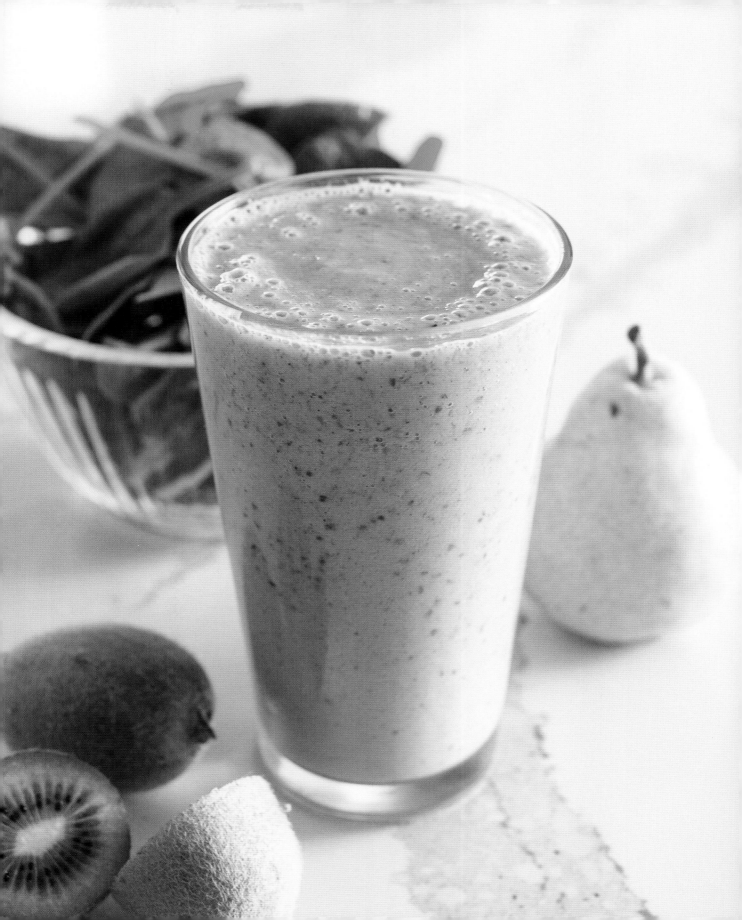

Strawberry Oatmeal Smoothie

Like a creamy bowl of oatmeal, this protein and fiber packed smoothie features sweet strawberries and banana for a quick post-workout meal replacement that'll keep you full and energized throughout the day.

Instructions:

1. Add all the ingredients into a blender and process on high speed for 1 to 2 minutes or until the mixture is smooth and creamy. Add a little water if you prefer a looser consistency.

2. Pour the smoothie into a glass and enjoy immediately.

Notes

Please be aware that any ingredient additions, omissions, or substitutions will affect the nutritional information.

- For a dairy-free option, substitute any nut milk of your choice for the full-fat cow's milk.
- When choosing a protein powder, use a high-quality, clean protein powder from grass-fed cows with no additives, fillers, gums, or anti-caking agents.
- For a vegetarian option, omit the protein powder.
- Make sure to use hulled tahini paste and not unhulled. Hulled tahini has had the outer shell removed from the seed and results in a milder flavor with the added benefit of higher absorption rates of calcium and other important minerals.
- You can substitute any nut butter of your choice, such as cashew, almond, or peanut, for the tahini paste.

Difficulty: **Easy**

High Protein | High Carb | Grain Free | Gluten Free | Vegetarian (optional) | Egg Free | Dairy Free (optional)

Prep Time | 5 minutes

Total Time | 5 minutes

Yield | 1 serving

Calories Per Serving | 514

Total Carbs | 51 g

Net Carbs | 43 g

Protein | 34 g

Fat | 19 g

Ingredients:

1 cup (235 ml) full-fat cow's milk (see notes)

1 tablespoon (15 g) tahini paste (hulled)

¼ cup (24 g) gluten-free rolled oats

½ frozen banana

1 cup (145 g) strawberries, washed and halved

1 scoop protein powder (optional)

1 teaspoon pure vanilla extract

Pinch of salt

Electrolyte Replenisher

This refreshing and hydrating drink is ideal to replenish your lost electrolytes after a sweaty session at the gym. Loaded with important salts and trace minerals and sweetened with tropical coconut water, nothing quenches your thirst better!

Instructions:

1. Add all the ingredients into a large drinking glass and stir until fully combined and the salts have dissolved. Serve immediately and enjoy.

Notes

Please be aware that any ingredient additions, omissions, or substitutions will affect the nutritional information.

- If you prefer it a little sweeter, simply add more honey or any natural sweetener of your choice.
- It's best to avoid ultra-processed sports drinks or supplements that are usually full of additives, hidden sugars, and fillers. However, a clean unflavored trace mineral salt supplement is a great addition to this recipe in place of the pink Himalayan or sea salt.

Difficulty: **Easy**

High Carb | Grain Free | Gluten Free | Vegetarian | Egg Free | Dairy Free

Prep Time | 5 minutes

Total Time | 5 minutes

Yield | 1 serving

Calories Per Serving | 90

Total Carbs | 22 g

Net Carbs | 19 g

Protein | 2 g

Fat | 0 g

Ingredients:

1 cup (235 ml) coconut water

1 cup (235 ml) water

2 teaspoons raw honey

½ teaspoon pink Himalayan or sea salt (see notes)

2 small limes, juiced

Chocolate Malt Collagen Shake

This rich and chocolatey shake is naturally sweet thanks to the fiber-rich banana and Medjool dates, and it's packed with gut healing collagen to help repair your muscles after an intense workout session.

Instructions:

1. Add all the ingredients into a blender and process on high speed for 1 to 2 minutes or until the mixture is smooth and creamy. Add a little water if you prefer a looser consistency.

2. Pour the smoothie into a glass and enjoy immediately.

Notes

Please be aware that any ingredient additions, omissions, or substitutions will affect the nutritional information.

- When choosing collagen powder, use a high-quality, clean collagen powder from grass-fed cows with no additives, fillers, gums, or anti-caking agents.

- If using bone broth, make sure it's unflavored in the cooking process so it doesn't throw off the sweetness in this recipe—I promise you won't even taste it! Use plain store-bought broth or if making your own, simply omit the vegetables, herbs, and spices in the cooking process.

- For a pescatarian option, replace the bone broth with any nut milk of your choice and substitute marine collagen for the bovine collagen powder.

- For a dairy-free option, substitute any nut milk of your choice for the full-fat cow's milk.

Difficulty: **Easy**

High Protein | High Carb | Grain Free | Gluten Free | Egg Free | Pescatarian (optional) | Dairy Free (optional)

Prep Time | 5 minutes

Total Time | 5 minutes

Yield | 1 serving

Calories Per Serving | 470

Total Carbs | 47 g

Net Carbs | 43 g

Protein | 28 g

Fat | 15 g

Ingredients:

¾ cup (175 ml) unflavored chicken bone broth (see notes)

¾ cup (175 ml) full-fat cow's milk (see notes)

1 tablespoon (16 g) cashew butter

½ frozen banana

1 Medjool date, pitted

1 scoop collagen powder

¼ teaspoon ground cinnamon

1 teaspoon raw cacao powder

Pinch of salt

3–4 ice cubes

Protein Brownies

Soft, gooey, and chewy, these healthy chocolate brownies are a carb-rich treat, perfect for your more intense workout days thanks to the natural sweetness of golden baked sweet potato and decadent dark chocolate.

Instructions:

1. Preheat the oven to 325°F (170°C, or gas mark 3) and place the rack in the middle of the oven. Line an 8 x 8-inch (20 x 20-cm) brownie pan with parchment paper.

2. If the almond butter is firm, melt over low heat in a small saucepan until soft and runny.

3. Transfer the almond butter to a large mixing bowl, add the sweet potato purée (or baked and cooled sweet potato flesh) and vanilla extract, and mix until fully incorporated.

4. Add the dry ingredients to the bowl and stir to combine. Add the chocolate chips and mix well.

5. Transfer the batter to the brownie pan and smooth down evenly with a spatula.

6. Bake in the oven 20 minutes. Remove from the oven and allow to cool fully for 20 to 30 minutes on a wire rack.

7. Cut into 16 slices, serve, and enjoy!

Notes

Please be aware that any ingredient additions, omissions, or substitutions will affect the nutritional information.

- If buying store-bought sweet potato purée, choose 100% pure sweet potato with no added sugars or preservatives.
- For a nut-free option, you can use any seed butter of your choice such sunflower seed butter.
- Brownies firm up once they cool, so they will look underdone when they come out of the oven. If you prefer them even firmer, cover and chill in the fridge a few hours before serving.
- Store in an airtight container in single layers separated by parchment paper in the fridge for up to a week.

Difficulty: **Easy**

High Protein | High Carb | Gluten Free | Vegetarian (optional) | Dairy Free | Egg Free | Nut Free (optional)

Prep Time | 15 minutes

Cook Time | 20 minutes

Total Time | 35 minutes

Yield | 16 brownies

Calories Per Brownie | 210

Total Carbs | 17 g

Net Carbs | 13 g

Protein | 10 g

Fat | 11 g

Ingredients:

1 cup (260 g) almond butter or any nut butter of your choice

1 cup (246 g) sweet potato purée or baked sweet potato

1 teaspoon pure vanilla extract

6 tablespoons (34 g) gluten-free oat flour

⅓ cup (40 g) vanilla protein powder (optional)

⅓ cup (48 g) coconut sugar

6 tablespoons (30 g) raw cacao powder

1½ teaspoons baking soda

Pinch of salt

½ cup (120 g) unsweetened dark chocolate chips

Coconut Energy Balls

Densely satisfying, sweet and nutty, these no-bake energy balls are superfast and easy to make. Full of fiber and protein, they're a great option when you feel like something sweet after your workout or when the afternoon slump hits!

Instructions:

1. Add all the ingredients into a food processor and blend until a dough forms. See notes below for tips on consistency.

2. Use a medium cookie scoop or your hands to grab dough and roll into 10 balls, even in size.

3. Transfer onto a baking sheet and chill in the fridge for 30 minutes before serving!

Notes

Please be aware that any ingredient additions, omissions, or substitutions will affect the nutritional information.

- When choosing a protein powder, use a high-quality, clean protein powder from grass-fed cows with no additives, fillers, gums, or anti-caking agents.
- For a vegetarian option, omit the protein powder.
- Soaking the dates beforehand will help soften them up so they combine easily with the other ingredients.
- If the mixture is too dry, add more sticky ingredients like dates, nut butter, raw honey, 100% pure maple syrup, or a dash of water.
- If the mixture is too wet, then add more protein powder or shredded coconut. A little almond flour may also help.
- Store in an airtight container in single layers separated by parchment paper in the fridge for up to 10 days.

Difficulty: **Easy**

High Protein | High Carb | Grain Free | Gluten Free | Vegetarian (optional) | Dairy Free | Egg Free

Prep Time | 5 minutes

Chill Time | 30 minutes

Total Time | 35 minutes

Yield | 10 energy balls

Calories Per Energy Ball | 189

Total Carbs | 12 g

Net Carbs | 8 g

Protein | 13 g

Fat | 10 g

Ingredients:

½ cup (130 g) almond butter or any nut butter of your choice

3 Medjool dates, soaked and pitted

⅓ cup (40 g) protein powder (optional)

¼ cup (20 g) unsweetened shredded coconut

1 tablespoon (13 g) chia seeds

½ teaspoon ground cinnamon

1 teaspoon pure vanilla extract

Pinch of salt

StrongCurves

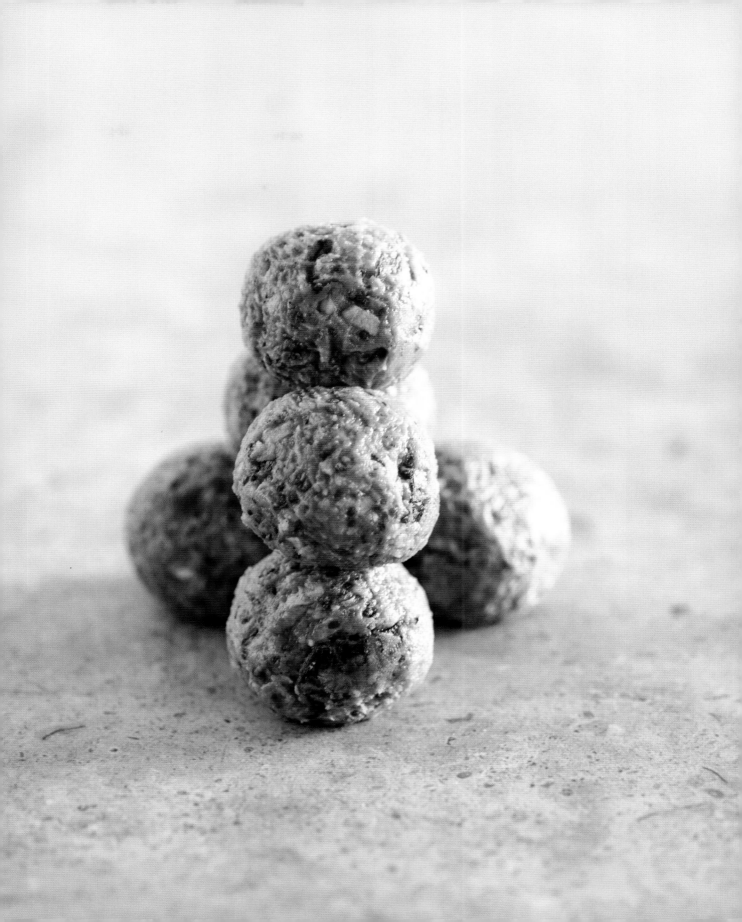

Honey Puffed Rice Bars

This nostalgic kid's treat was always a winner in my packed school lunches. But with all the added sugars and processed ingredients, it definitely wasn't a healthy choice! Which is why this reimagined healthy version is so much better. Full of healthy fats, fiber, and the natural sweetness of honey, these crispy rice bars are a great sweet option for your post-workout snack.

Instructions:

1. Line an 8 x 8-inch (20 x 20-cm) pan with parchment paper and set aside.

2. Melt the cashew butter, coconut oil, honey, and vanilla extract in a medium saucepan over low heat. Mix until smooth and well combined, about 1 minute. Remove from the heat and add the protein powder and puffed rice cereal. Stir until fully incorporated.

3. Pour the puffed rice mixture into the pan and use a spatula to evenly level out the mixture. Chill in the fridge for 30 minutes or until the bars are set.

4. Sprinkle with salt and then cut into 16 bars. Enjoy!

Notes

Please be aware that any ingredient additions, omissions, or substitutions will affect the nutritional information.

- You can use any nut butter of your choice such as almond or peanut butter.
- You can use any sticky sweetener of your choice such as 100% pure maple syrup or brown rice syrup.
- When choosing a protein powder, use a high-quality, clean protein powder from grass-fed cows with no additives, fillers, gums, or anti-caking agents.
- For a vegetarian option, omit the protein powder.
- Store in an airtight container in single layers separated by parchment paper in the fridge for up to a week.

Difficulty: **Easy**

High Protein | High Carb | Gluten Free | Vegetarian (optional) | Dairy Free | Egg Free

Prep Time | 5 minutes

Cook Time | 5 minutes

Chill Time | 30 minutes

Total Time | 40 minutes

Yield | 16 bars

Calories Per Bar | 158

Total Carbs | 14 g

Net Carbs | 13 g

Protein | 8 g

Fat | 9 g

Ingredients:

¾ cup (195 g) cashew butter

2 tablespoons (28 g) coconut oil

⅓ cup (115 g) raw honey

1 teaspoon pure vanilla extract

½ cup (60 g) vanilla protein powder (optional)

3 cups (51 g) puffed rice cereal

Pinch of salt

Protein-Packed Chocolate Pudding

With only four ingredients, this creamy and rich chocolate pudding is surprisingly high in protein thanks to its secret ingredient—blended cottage cheese! Enjoy as a treat when the sweet tooth hits, especially after a heavy weights session.

Instructions:

1. Add all the ingredients into a food processor and blend for 1 to 2 minutes until smooth and creamy.

2. Spoon the mixture into a mason jar and chill in the fridge for 1 to 2 hours before serving.

Notes

Please be aware that any ingredient additions, omissions, or substitutions will affect the nutritional information.

- When choosing a protein powder, use a high-quality, clean protein powder from grass-fed cows with no additives, fillers, gums, or anti-caking agents.

- For a vegetarian option, omit the protein powder.

- For a low-carb version, substitute an equivalent amount of keto-friendly sweetener, such as stevia, monk fruit, or powdered erythritol, for the raw honey.

Difficulty: **Easy**

High Protein | Grain Free | Gluten Free | Vegetarian (optional) | Egg Free | Nut Free

Prep Time | 5 minutes

Chill Time | 2 hours

Total Time | 2 hours, 5 minutes

Yield | 6 servings

Calories Per Serving | 192

Total Carbs | 10 g

Net Carbs | 9 g

Protein | 18 g

Fat | 7 g

Ingredients:

16 ounces (455 g) full-fat cottage cheese

⅔ cup (53 g) raw cacao powder

3 scoops vanilla protein powder (optional)

2 tablespoons (40 g) raw honey

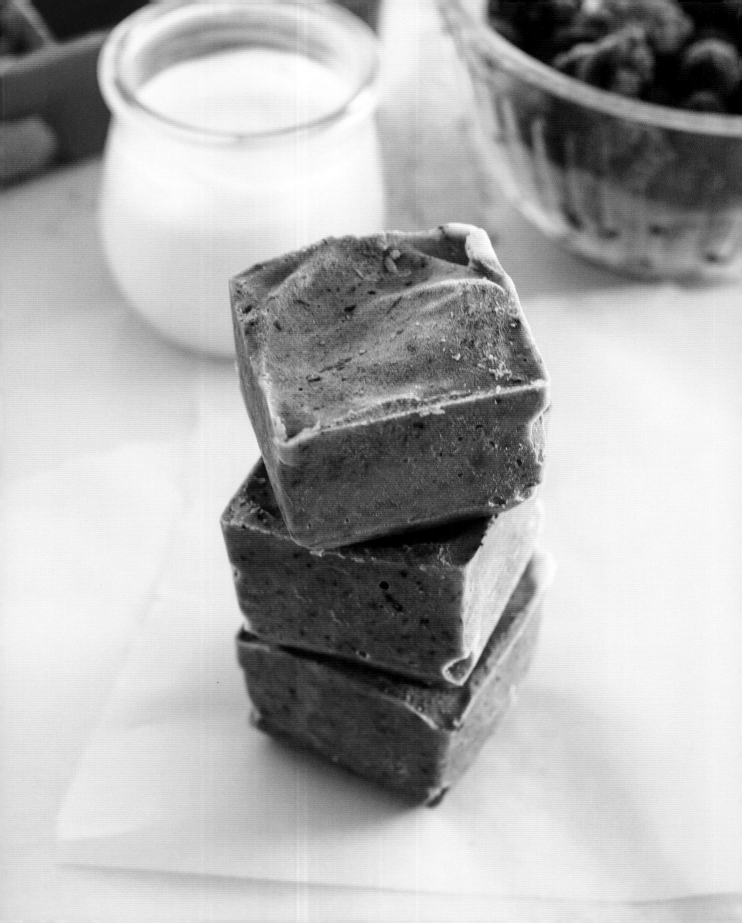

Frozen Yogurt Bites

So simple, yet so creamy and delicious, with only three ingredients, these fruity frozen yogurt bites are an easy high-protein snack post-workout.

Instructions:

1. Add all the ingredients into a food processor and blend for 1 to 2 minutes until smooth and creamy.

2. Spoon the mixture into small silicone molds and set in the freezer for a minimum of 3 hours before serving.

Notes

Please be aware that any ingredient additions, omissions, or substitutions will affect the nutritional information.

- For a dairy-free option, substitute plain or vanilla coconut yogurt for the Greek yogurt.
- When choosing a protein powder, use a high-quality, clean protein powder from grass-fed cows with no additives, fillers, gums, or anti-caking agents.
- For a vegetarian option, omit the protein powder.
- Yogurt bites can be stored in a zip top bag in the freezer for up to 3 months.

Difficulty: **Easy**

High Protein | Grain Free | Gluten Free | Vegetarian (optional) | Dairy Free (optional) | Egg Free | Nut Free

Prep Time | 5 minutes

Chill Time | 3 hours

Total Time | 3 hours, 5 minutes

Yield | 8 yogurt bites

Calories Per Yogurt Bite | 107

Total Carbs | 6 g

Net Carbs | 5 g

Protein | 9 g

Fat | 5 g

Ingredients:

12 ounces (340 g) full-fat Greek yogurt (see notes)

3 scoops vanilla protein powder (optional)

1 cup (163 g) frozen mixed berries

3

Rest Days

High Protein + Higher Fats + Lower Carbs

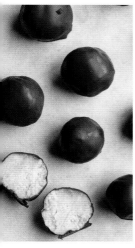

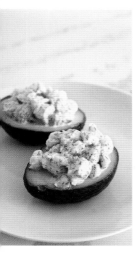

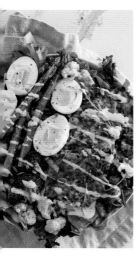

Whether you prefer to take the whole day off and relax at home or stay slightly active by doing some gentle yoga or light cardio, rest days are about caring for the body, rather than stressing it. It's a day for recovery and replenishment, so it's important to give your body the nutrients it needs in order to repair and rebuild your muscles after the previous day's workout. High protein meals with healthy fats are ideal because they contain all the amino acids your muscles need to grow from the protein, while the healthy fats support your hormones and nervous system. But remember, because your activity levels are lower, you really don't need to load up with high-energy, carb-heavy meals. Stick to gut-healthy fiber such as leafy greens and veggies, nuts, and seeds instead of starchy foods like potatoes or rice.

You may find that you feel hungrier the day after an intense lifting session because your body is actually working overtime on the inside to help your muscles rebuild and your nervous system adapt. So, even if you're on a scheduled rest day, it's important to still eat enough and honor your hunger. Skipping meals, restricting calories, or feeling like you haven't "earned" the right to eat because you haven't exercised on your day off are unhealthy thoughts that will hinder your progress. Remember, your body knows best. Listen to her, and she'll thrive.

Grain-Free Porridge

A creamy high-fiber porridge made with almond flour and topped with berries makes this a nourishing and filling rest day breakfast.

Instructions:

1. Add the flaxseed meal, almond flour, and collagen or protein powder to a small saucepan over low heat and stir to combine. Add the milk to the saucepan and turn heat up to medium. Cook for 1 to 2 minutes, stirring constantly, until warmed and thick in consistency. Add more milk if it's too thick.

2. Transfer to a serving bowl, drizzle with honey, top with blueberries, and serve!

Notes

Please be aware that any ingredient additions, omissions, or substitutions will affect the nutritional information.

- When choosing a collagen or protein powder, use a high-quality, clean powder from grass-fed cows with no additives, fillers, gums, or anti-caking agents.
- For a vegetarian option, omit the collagen or protein powder.
- For a dairy-free option, substitute any nut milk of your choice for the full-fat cow's milk.
- For a keto-friendly option, substitute an equivalent amount of keto-friendly sweetener, such as stevia, monk fruit, or erythritol, for the raw honey.

Difficulty: Easy

High Protein | Low Carb | Grain Free | Gluten Free | Vegetarian (optional) | Egg Free | Dairy Free (optional) | Keto Friendly (optional)

Prep Time | 2 minutes

Cook Time | 2 minutes

Total Time | 4 minutes

Yield | 1 serving

Calories Per Serving | 503

Total Carbs | 33 g

Net Carbs | 23 g

Protein | 35 g

Fat | 26 g

Ingredients:

- 3 tablespoons (21 g) flaxseed meal (linseed)
- 3 tablespoons (21 g) almond flour
- 1 scoop unflavored collagen or protein powder (optional)
- ¾ cup (175 ml) full-fat cow's milk (see notes)
- 1 teaspoon raw honey or 100% pure maple syrup
- ¼ cup (36 g) fresh blueberries

Avo Egg Smash

Here's a no-fuss easy breakfast that's packed full of protein and healthy fats. It may not look so pretty, but it's oh-so satisfying and will keep your hunger at bay until lunch.

Instructions:

1. Fill a medium saucepan with water and bring to a rolling boil over high heat. Carefully add the eggs to the boiling water and set timer for 4 to 5 minutes for runny eggs or 6 to 7 minutes for soft-boiled eggs.

2. While the eggs are boiling, cut an avocado lengthwise and scoop the flesh of one side into a bowl. Roughly mash avocado with a fork and season with salt, pepper, and chile flakes to taste.

3. As soon as timer goes off, run the eggs under cold water for a few minutes before peeling.

4. Top the smashed avocado with the soft-boiled eggs and enjoy!

Difficulty: **Easy**

Vegetarian | Strict Low Carb | Gluten Free | Grain Free | Dairy Free | Nut Free

Prep Time | 5 minutes

Cook Time | 7 minutes

Total Time | 12 minutes

Yield | 1 serving

Calories Per Serving | 339

Total Carbs | 9 g

Net Carbs | 3 g

Protein | 21 g

Fat | 25 g

Ingredients:

3 large pasture-raised eggs, room temperature

½ large avocado

½ teaspoon pink Himalayan rock salt or sea salt

¼ teaspoon black pepper

Pinch of chile flakes (optional)

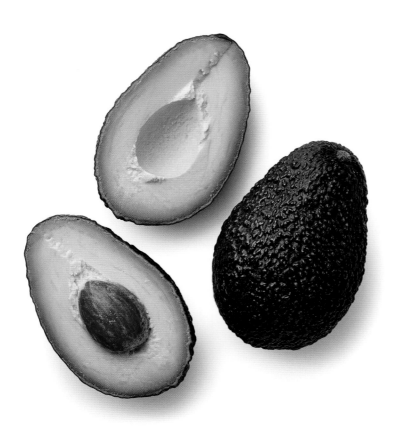

Salmon and Cream Cheese Sushi

Have you ever wanted to have sushi for breakfast? Now you can! These creamy avocado-filled smoked salmon rolls boast healthy fats and satiating protein, but omit the carbs you'd normally get from the sushi rice. It's the perfect way to enjoy the experience of sushi without the rice-induced crash, while nourishing your body on your rest day.

Instructions:

1. Place a large piece of plastic wrap on your work surface. You can also use a sushi roller.

2. Overlap the salmon slices on the plastic wrap to make a rectangle roughly 6 x 12-inch (15 x 30-cm) long, with one of the longest sides facing you.

3. Spread the cream cheese over the salmon carefully without moving the salmon slices out of place.

4. Place the cucumber and avocado along one side of the rectangle closest to you, about ½ inch (1.3 cm) from the edge. Sprinkle them with sesame seeds.

5. Using the plastic wrap as a guide, roll the salmon up tightly around the filling.

6. Chill in the fridge for 30 minutes or until firm.

7. Using a sharp knife, cut the roll into 12 pieces. Serve with a squeeze of lemon.

Difficulty: **Moderate**

High Protein | Low Carb | Grain Free | Gluten Free | Pescatarian | Egg Free | Nut Free

Prep Time | 10 minutes

Chill Time | 30 minutes

Total Time | 40 minutes

Yield | 4 servings (12 pieces)

Calories Per Serving | 407

Total Carbs | 5 g

Net Carbs | 3 g

Protein | 31 g

Fat | 30 g

Ingredients:

16 ounces (455 g) smoked salmon

½ cup (115 g) full-fat cream cheese

½ cucumber, peeled and thinly sliced lengthwise

½ large avocado, thinly sliced

1 teaspoon sesame seeds

½ tablespoon lemon juice (optional)

Egg and Feta Muffins

Pairing eggs with creamy feta, juicy tomatoes, and fresh spinach make this a healthy "grab and go" option that you can whip up in minutes.

Instructions:

1. Preheat the oven to 350°F (180°C, or gas mark 4) and place the rack in the middle of the oven. Grease a muffin pan or line with silicone muffin liners.

2. Beat the eggs in a large mixing bowl and add the spinach, cherry tomatoes, salt, and pepper. Mix to combine.

3. Evenly pour the mixture into the muffin pan and top each cup with the feta cheese.

4. Bake for 15 to 18 minutes or until fluffy and golden. Remove from the oven and let cool for a few minutes on wire cooling rack.

5. Garnish with chives and serve.

Notes

Please be aware that any ingredient additions, omissions, or substitutions will affect the nutritional information.

For a dairy-free option, simply omit the feta cheese.

Difficulty: **Easy**

High Protein | Low Carb | Grain Free | Gluten Free | Vegetarian | Nut Free | Dairy Free (optional)

Prep Time | 5 minutes

Cook Time | 20 minutes

Total Time | 25 minutes

Yield | 3 servings (12 muffins)

Calories Per Serving | 279

Total Carbs | 3 g

Net Carbs | 2 g

Protein | 23 g

Fat | 18 g

Ingredients:

10 large pasture-raised eggs

½ cup (22 g) baby spinach, finely chopped

6 cherry tomatoes, diced

½ teaspoon salt

¼ teaspoon black pepper

¼ cup (38 g) feta cheese, crumbled (optional)

1 teaspoon chopped chives

Grain-Free Granola

This healthier low-sugar twist on the popular breakfast staple is ideal on days when your activity levels are low. High in protein and healthy fats to keep cravings at bay, this crunchy granola is also great as a midafternoon snack on its own.

Instructions:

1. Preheat the oven to 325°F (170°C, or gas mark 3) and place the rack in the top third of the oven. Line a baking sheet with parchment paper.

2. In a small saucepan, melt the butter over low heat. Set aside to cool slightly, about 5 minutes. When cooled, add the egg white, honey, and vanilla and stir to combine.

3. In a large mixing bowl add the mixed nuts, flaxseed meal, sunflower seeds, pepitas, cinnamon, and salt and stir to combine.

4. Pour the melted butter mixture into the bowl of dry ingredients and mix well to combine.

5. Spread the granola mixture evenly on the baking sheet and bake in the oven for 7 to 8 minutes until the edges are golden—do not overbake!

6. Remove from the oven and allow to cool fully so the granola hardens. Then, break up into chunks and store in an airtight container.

7. Add the yogurt to a serving bowl, top with a portion of granola and berries, and serve.

Notes

Please be aware that any ingredient additions, omissions, or substitutions will affect the nutritional information.

- For a dairy-free option, substitute an equivalent amount of coconut oil for the grass-fed butter and serve with coconut yogurt instead of Greek yogurt.

- For a keto-friendly option, substitute an equivalent amount of keto-friendly sweetener, such as stevia, monk fruit, or erythritol, for the raw honey.

Difficulty: **Easy**

High Protein | Low Carb | Grain Free | Gluten Free | Vegetarian | Dairy Free (optional) | Keto Friendly (optional)

Prep Time | 5 minutes

Cook Time | 8 minutes

Total Time | 13 minutes

Yield | 10 servings

Calories Per Serving | 616

Total Carbs | 31 g

Net Carbs | 23 g

Protein | 31 g

Fat | 44 g

Ingredients:

FOR THE GRANOLA:

3½ tablespoons (49 g) grass-fed butter, melted (see notes)

1 pasture-raised egg white

1 tablespoon (20 g) raw honey (see notes)

1 teaspoon pure vanilla extract

3 cups (435 g) raw mixed nuts, coarsely chopped

½ cup (56 g) flaxseed meal (linseed)

⅓ cup (48 g) sunflower seeds

⅓ cup (47 g) pepitas

1 teaspoon ground cinnamon

¼ teaspoon salt

FOR SERVING:

1 cup (230 g) full-fat Greek yogurt (see notes)

½ cup (70 g) fresh berries

Blueberry Breakfast Bake

If this recipe sounds familiar to you, you're not wrong—it's a recovery day take on the Apricot Breakfast Bake (page 72). This version is lower in carbs and loaded with healthy fats for those days when the order of the day is to rest and recoup.

Instructions:

1. Preheat the oven to 375°F (190°C, or gas mark 5) and place the rack in the middle of the oven. Line an 8 x 8-inch (20 x 20-cm) baking dish with parchment paper.

2. In a large bowl, add the blueberries, erythritol, and lemon juice and stir to combine. Transfer the blueberry mixture to the baking dish and spread it evenly along the bottom of the dish with a spatula.

3. In a separate mixing bowl, combine the almond flour, coconut flour, protein powder, 2 tablespoons (14 g) of pecans, baking powder, cinnamon, and salt. Mix well to combine.

4. Sprinkle the almond flour mixture evenly over the top of the blueberry mixture to cover fully. Then, drizzle the melted butter over the top to coat the almond flour mixture.

5. Sprinkle the remaining pecans on top and bake for 30 to 35 minutes until the crust has browned and the blueberries are bubbly. Remove from the oven and let cool for 5 minutes before serving.

Notes

Please be aware that any ingredient additions, omissions, or substitutions will affect the nutritional information.

- For a dairy-free option, use coconut oil in place of the grass-fed butter.
- This recipe is keto friendly, but if you prefer using natural sweeteners, use coconut sugar instead of erythritol; however, the carb count will be much higher.
- When choosing a protein powder, use a high-quality, clean protein powder from grass-fed cows with no additives, fillers, gums, or anti-caking agents.

Difficulty: **Easy**

High Protein | Low Carb | Grain Free | Gluten Free | Egg Free | Dairy Free (optional)

Prep Time | 15 minutes

Cook Time | 35 minutes

Total Time | 50 minutes

Yield | 6 servings

Calories Per Serving | 409

Total Carbs | 24 g

Net Carbs | 16 g

Protein | 23 g

Fat | 25 g

Ingredients:

3 cups (465 g) frozen blueberries

½ cup (96 g) erythritol or sweetener of your choice

1 tablespoon (15 ml) lemon juice

¼ cup (28 g) almond flour

½ cup (56 g) coconut flour

½ cup (60 g) protein powder

¼ cup (28 g) chopped pecans, divided

1 teaspoon baking powder

1 teaspoon ground cinnamon

½ teaspoon salt

½ cup (112 g) unsalted grass-fed butter, melted (see notes)

Shrimp-Stuffed Avocado

A deconstructed shrimp cocktail with creamy avocado and juicy shrimp makes this a quick and easy lunch recipe. Full of healthy fats and protein, it's got everything you need for a nourishing and fuss-free rest day lunch.

Instructions:

1. Add the shrimp, mayonnaise, dill, salt, and pepper into a small mixing bowl. Mix well to combine.

2. Spoon half the mixture into the hollow of each avocado and serve.

Notes

Please be aware that any ingredient additions, omissions, or substitutions will affect the nutritional information.

- For a vegetarian option, substitute 2 boiled eggs for the tiger shrimp.
- When buying store-bought mayonnaise, look for high-quality brands that use olive oil or avocado oil rather than vegetable or seed oils and avoid preservatives and additives. Or use your favorite recipe to make your own homemade mayonnaise!

Difficulty: **Easy**

Low Carb | High Protein | Pescatarian | Vegetarian (optional) | Gluten Free | Grain Free | Nut Free

Prep Time | 5 minutes

Total Time | 5 minutes

Yield | 2 servings

Calories Per Serving | 293

Total Carbs | 10 g

Net Carbs | 4 g

Protein | 27 g

Fat | 18 g

Ingredients:

10 precooked tiger shrimp, peeled, deveined, and chopped (see notes)

2 tablespoons (28 g) olive oil mayonnaise

1 tablespoon (4 g) chopped fresh dill

½ teaspoon salt

¼ teaspoon black pepper

1 large avocado, halved lengthwise and pit removed

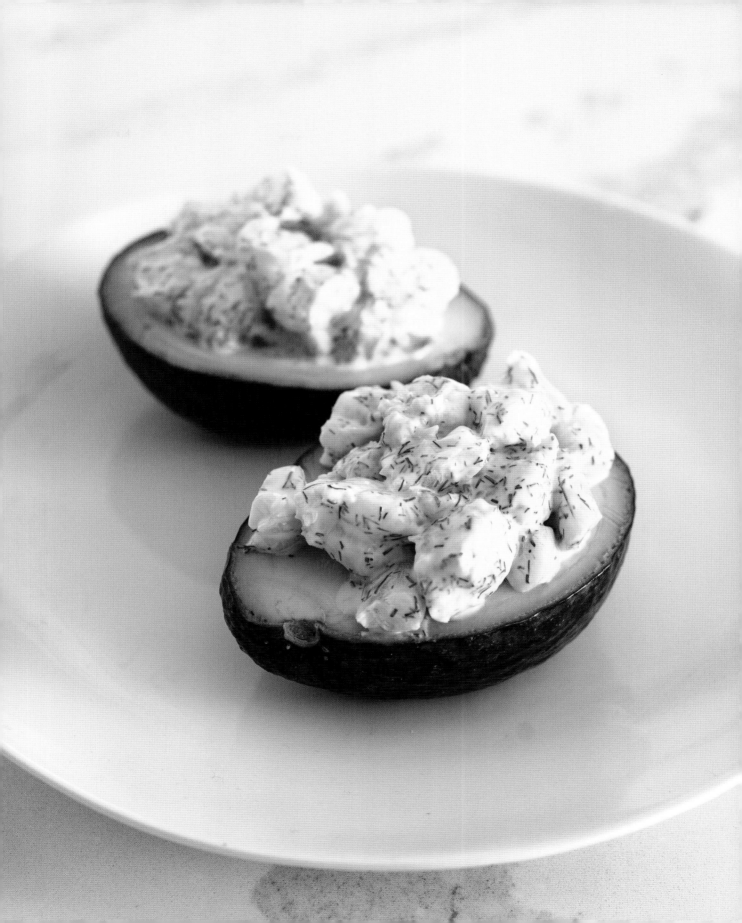

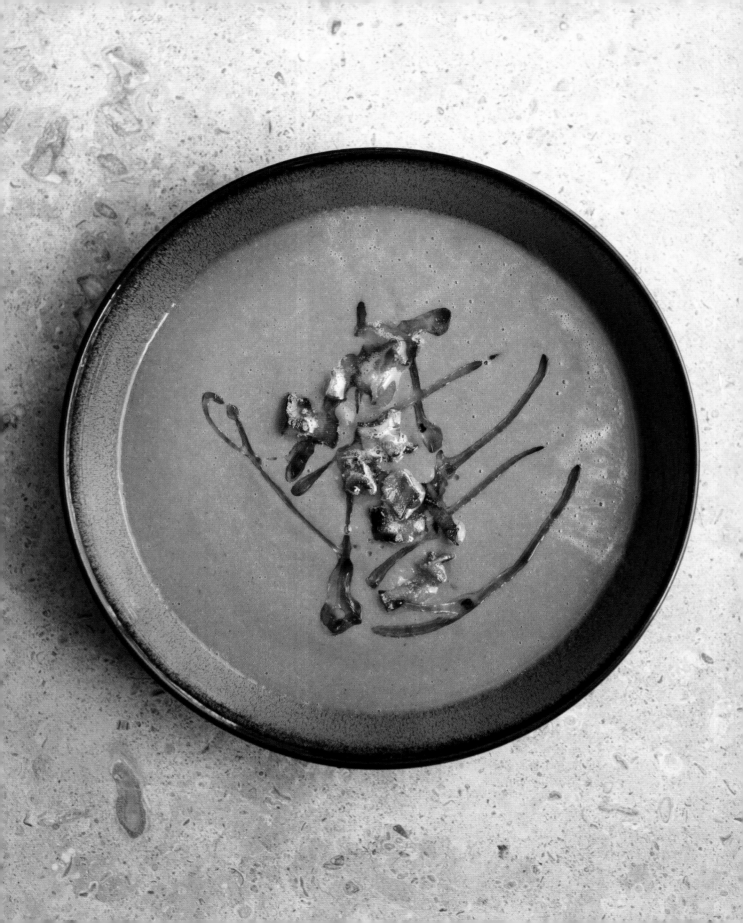

Mushroom and Bacon Soup

Creamy mushrooms, aromatic herbs, and nourishing broth make this hearty soup a perfect winter rest day meal, with plenty of protein and healthy fats.

Instructions:

1. Finely chop the bacon and fry in a skillet over medium heat until crispy. Remove from the heat and transfer the bacon to a paper towel-lined plate to drain.

2. Heat the butter in a stock pot or large saucepan over medium heat. Add the onion and garlic and sauté for a few minutes until soft and translucent. Add the mushrooms to the pot along with the thyme, parsley, salt, and pepper. Sauté until the mushrooms cook down and release their liquid, about 5 minutes. Add the chicken bone broth and cream to the pot and bring to a boil. Then, lower the heat to a simmer for 30 minutes, stirring occasionally.

3. Transfer the soup to a blender (or use an immersion blender) and pulse until smooth. Do this in two batches so the liquid doesn't spill out of your blender.

4. Divide the soup between four bowls, drizzle with a dash of olive oil, top with the bacon, and serve!

Notes

Make the Healing Bone Broth (page 166) ahead of time to use in this recipe. Alternatively, you can buy premade bone broth or stock, but make sure it's from pasture-raised high-quality chicken bones.

Difficulty: **Easy**

Strict Low Carb | Gluten Free | Grain Free | Egg Free | Nut Free

Prep Time | 10 minutes

Cook Time | 30 minutes

Total Time | 40 minutes

Yield | 4 servings

Calories Per Serving | 340

Total Carbs | 8 g

Net Carbs | 6 g

Protein | 20 g

Fat | 18 g

Ingredients:

2 slices center-cut bacon

1 tablespoon (14 g) grass-fed butter

½ yellow onion, diced

1 garlic clove, minced

4 cups (280 g) white or brown mushrooms, roughly chopped

1 teaspoon dried thyme

2 tablespoons (8 g) chopped fresh parsley

1 teaspoon pink Himalayan rock salt or sea salt

¼ teaspoon black pepper

4 cups (946 ml) Healing Bone Broth (page 166) or store-bought chicken bone broth or stock (see notes)

⅓ cup (80 ml) heavy cream

1 teaspoon olive oil

Salmon and Cream Cheese Crepes

These protein-packed fluffy crepes feature a smoked salmon, cream cheese, and dill filling for a healthier twist on the popular lox bagel. Minus the extra carbs, they'll leave you satisfied, but feeling light.

Instructions:

1. Prepare the crepes in advance and store in an airtight container in the fridge until ready to use.

2. To make the crepe batter, add all the crepe ingredients to a food processor and pulse until fully incorporated and a loose batter forms.

3. Heat a little butter in a skillet over medium heat and ladle the batter in, swirling it around to evenly distribute.

4. Cook until the top is firm, about 2 minutes. Flip and fry the other side, another 2 to 3 minutes. Remove from the heat and let cool on a paper towel-lined plate.

5. Repeat with the remaining batter, wiping the pan clean after each time and using a little more butter as needed.

6. To assemble the crepe, spoon the cream cheese into the center, top with the smoked salmon, dill, and capers. Roll up the crepe and serve immediately.

Notes

This recipe calls for psyllium husks, not psyllium husk powder. If using the latter, use half the amount shown in the recipe. Psyllium is a soluble fiber used in gluten-free baking for its binding properties and can be found in most health food stores and online.

Difficulty: **Moderate**

Low Carb | High Protein | Pescatarian | Gluten Free | Grain Free

Prep Time | 5 minutes

Cook Time | 18 minutes

Total Time | 23 minutes

Yield | 6 crepes

Calories Per Serving | 485

Total Carbs | 21 g

Net Carbs | 9 g

Protein | 43 g

Fat | 31 g

Ingredients:

FOR THE CREPES:

4 whole large pasture-raised eggs

4 large pasture-raised eggs, whites only

2 tablespoons (10 g) psyllium husk (see notes)

½ cup (115 g) full-fat cream cheese

Unsalted grass-fed butter, for frying

FOR THE FILLING:

1 tablespoon (15 g) full-fat cream cheese

3½ ounces (98 g) smoked salmon

1 tablespoon (4 g) chopped fresh dill

1 teaspoon capers, drained

Zucchini Fritters with Fried Eggs

A healthier take on a staple Aussie cafe brunch, these fritters are packed with fiber and topped with gooey fried eggs for a delicious protein-filled breakfast.

Instructions:

1. Place the zucchini in a large mixing bowl and add the basil, almond flour, egg, garlic powder, paprika, and salt and mix well until combined. Using a tablespoon or cookie scoop, divide the mixture into balls (about 8), flatten them down into disc shapes, and transfer to a plate.

2. Heat a little coconut oil in a large skillet over medium-high heat. Add 4 fritters to the skillet at a time and fry, flipping them over when golden, about 3 to 5 minutes each side. Remove from the heat and set aside on a paper towel-lined plate.

3. Repeat with the rest of the fritters. Clean the pan with a paper towel as you go and add more coconut oil as needed. To avoid burning, do not overcrowd the pan.

4. Wipe the skillet clean and add a little more coconut oil. Crack the eggs into the skillet and lower to medium heat. Cook for 3 to 5 minutes until the whites have cooked through. Flip and cook for another minute. Remove from the heat.

5. Divide the zucchini fritters on to 2 plates, top with 2 eggs on each plate, garnish with chives and chile flakes, and serve.

Notes

- Removing as much excess liquid as possible from the zucchinis before cooking will make sure your fritters don't turn out soggy. The best way to do this is to shred the zucchini using the smallest holes on a box grater and then place the zucchini in a cheesecloth or clean paper towel and squeeze the liquid out.

- Fritters can be made in advance and stored in an airtight container in the fridge for up to a week. To reheat, place on a baking sheet and heat in the oven on 300°F (150°C, or gas mark 2) for 10 minutes until warmed through.

Difficulty: **Moderate**

Low Carb | High Protein | Vegetarian | Gluten Free | Grain Free | Nut Free

Prep Time | 5 minutes

Cook Time | 10 minutes

Total Time | 15 minutes

Yield | 2 servings (8 fritters)

Calories Per Serving | 397

Total Carbs | 12 g

Net Carbs | 7 g

Protein | 23 g

Fat | 30 g

Ingredients:

FOR THE FRITTERS:

2 large zucchinis, grated and drained (see notes)

1 tablespoon (3 g) chopped fresh basil

6 tablespoons (42 g) almond flour

1 large pasture-raised egg

¼ teaspoon garlic powder

1 teaspoon paprika

½ teaspoon salt

Coconut oil, for frying

FOR THE TOPPING:

4 large pasture-raised eggs

2 teaspoons chopped chives

Pinch of chile flakes

Mini Salmon Broccoli Quiche

A perfect bite-sized combo of creamy eggs, salmon, and broccoli makes for an easy on-the-go lunch.

Instructions:

1. Preheat the oven to 325°F (170°C, or gas mark 3) and place the rack in the middle of the oven. Grease a muffin pan or line with silicone muffin liners.

2. Season the salmon fillet with salt and pepper and place in the center of a square of parchment paper. Make a baking parcel for the salmon by bringing two sides of the parchment paper together over the fillet and folding them down together, leaving a pocket for the fillet inside. Then, fold the other two sides in to seal the parcel and place on a baking sheet. Bake in the oven for 12 to 15 minutes or until cooked through.

3. Remove the salmon from the oven and flake the fillet with a fork into a small mixing bowl. Set aside.

4. To make the base, add almond flour, butter, 1 egg, salt, and pepper to a mixing bowl and stir well to combine.

5. Divide the dough evenly into 12 balls and press each one into the muffin cups, around the base and up the sides. Prick with a fork and bake for 12 to 15 minutes until golden.

6. Remove from the oven and let cool on a wire rack.

7. To make the filling, whisk 3 eggs in a separate mixing bowl. Add the broccoli, flaked salmon, and dill and mix to combine.

8. Evenly pour the egg mixture into the baked crusts and bake in the oven for 15 to 20 minutes or until fluffy and golden. Remove from the oven and let cool on a wire rack for 5 minutes before serving.

Difficulty: **Moderate**

Low Carb | High Protein | Pescatarian | Gluten Free | Grain Free | Dairy Free (optional)

Prep Time | 15 minutes

Cook Time | 35 minutes

Total Time | 50 minutes

Yield | 3 servings (12 quiches)

Calories Per Serving | 417

Total Carbs | 4 g

Net Carbs | 2 g

Protein | 23 g

Fat | 34 g

Ingredients:

1 salmon fillet (7 ounces, or 200 g)

½ teaspoon salt, divided

¼ teaspoon black pepper, divided

1 cup (112 g) almond flour

2 ounces (55 g) grass-fed butter, melted (see notes)

4 large pasture-raised eggs

½ cup (36 g) finely chopped broccoli

1 tablespoon (4 g) chopped fresh dill

Cheesy Chicken Patties

These deliciously cheesy and gooey chicken patties are low in carbs, but loaded with healthy fats and protein. Paired with a crunchy salad or simply enjoyed on their own, they make an ideal rest day lunch.

Instructions:

1. Line a large baking sheet or cookie sheet with parchment paper.

2. In a large mixing bowl, add the ground chicken, cheddar cheese, almond flour, egg, garlic, dill, salt, pepper, and chile flakes and mix well to combine.

3. Scoop ½ cup (115 g) of the chicken mixture and form into a small patty using your hands. Repeat with the rest of the mixture. You should have 12 patties. Transfer the patties to the baking sheet and chill for 1 hour in the fridge.

4. Heat a little olive oil on a large skillet over medium heat. When the oil is hot, add 4 to 6 of the chicken patties, depending on how many fit. Cook about 3 to 5 minutes per side until cooked through and golden brown.

5. Transfer the patties to a paper towel-lined plate and repeat with the remaining patties. You may need to wipe the skillet clean with a paper towel and add a little more oil in between batches.

Notes

Chicken patties can be stored in an airtight container in the fridge for up to 5 days. They can be eaten cold with leftovers, added to salads, or reheated in the oven at 300°F (150°C, or gas mark 2) for 15 minutes.

Difficulty: Moderate

Low Carb | High Protein | Gluten Free | Grain Free

Prep Time	15 minutes
Chill Time	1 hour
Cook Time	35 minutes
Total Time	1 hour, 50 minutes
Yield	6 servings (12 patties)
Calories Per Serving	395
Total Carbs	4 g
Net Carbs	3 g
Protein	35 g
Fat	28 g

Ingredients:

2 pounds (900 g) ground chicken

1 cup (115 g) shredded cheddar cheese

½ cup (56 g) almond flour

1 large pasture-raised egg

2 garlic cloves, minced

2 teaspoons chopped dill

1 teaspoon salt

1 teaspoon black pepper

¼ teaspoon chile flakes, or more to taste

Olive oil, for frying

Baked Spinach and Feta Tortilla

Indulge in the flavors of Greece with this savory low-carb lunch, packed with protein-rich eggs, iron-rich spinach, and creamy feta cheese.

Instructions:

1. Preheat the oven to 400°F (200°C, or gas mark 6) and place the rack in the middle of the oven. Line a 10 x 7-inch (25 x 18-cm) baking dish with parchment paper. The dish should be slightly smaller than the tortilla, and the parchment paper should exceed the height of the dish.

2. Heat a little olive oil in a skillet over medium heat and sauté the green onion until softened, about one minute. Add the spinach and cook until wilted, about a minute. Add the salt, pepper, and dill and stir to combine. Remove the pan from the heat. Transfer the veggies to a paper towel-lined plate and pat dry to remove any excess liquid.

3. Press the tortilla into the center of the baking dish so that the edges come up the side of the dish. Crack the eggs on top of the tortilla and season with salt and pepper to taste. Spread the spinach mixture over the eggs and sprinkle the sun-dried tomatoes and feta and mozzarella cheeses on top.

4. Bake for 20 minutes or until the cheese is golden and bubbly and eggs are set to your desired doneness. Remove from the oven and let cool for a few minutes. Then, lift the tortilla out of the dish by the parchment paper.

5. Sprinkle with chile flakes, slice into four equals servings. And enjoy!

Difficulty: **Easy**

Low Carb | High Protein | Gluten Free | Grain Free | Nut Free | Vegetarian

Prep Time | 10 minutes

Cook Time | 20 minutes

Total Time | 30 minutes

Yield | 2 servings

Calories Per Serving | 331

Total Carbs | 20 g

Net Carbs | 11 g

Protein | 24 g

Fat | 19 g

Ingredients:

Olive oil, for cooking

1 tablespoon (6 g) chopped green onion

1 cup (43 g) chopped baby spinach

¼ teaspoon salt

¼ teaspoon black pepper

2 tablespoons (8 g) chopped fresh dill

1 large gluten-free tortilla

¼ cup (14 g) sun-dried tomatoes

3 large pasture-raised eggs

1 ounce (28 g) feta cheese, crumbled

½ cup (60 g) shredded mozzarella cheese

¼ teaspoon chile flakes (optional)

Pork Egg Roll in a Bowl

Craving the flavors of an egg roll but looking for a healthier alternative? Look no further than this delicious deconstructed "egg roll in a bowl." With ground pork, colorful crispy veggies, and flavorful seasonings, this dish is high in protein and healthy fats yet lower in carbs—perfect for a recovery day dinner.

Instructions:

1. Heat a little avocado oil in a large wok or skillet over medium-high heat. Add the onion and garlic and sauté until soft and translucent, about 2 to 3 minutes.

2. Add the ground pork and cook for 2 to 3 minutes, breaking it up with a wooden spoon so it browns evenly.

3. Add the coconut aminos, arrowroot powder, grated ginger, ground ginger, onion powder, chile flakes, salt, and pepper. Stir to combine and cook for another few minutes until fragrant.

4. Add the red and green cabbage and carrot and sauté until tender, about 5 minutes.

5. Divide into 2 serving bowls, garnish with sesame seeds and green onion, and serve.

Difficulty: Easy

Low Carb | High Protein | Gluten Free | Grain Free | Dairy Free | Nut Free

Prep Time | 10 minutes

Cook Time | 20 minutes

Total Time | 30 minutes

Yield | 2 servings

Calories Per Serving | 485

Total Carbs | 24 g

Net Carbs | 22 g

Protein | 36 g

Fat | 30 g

Ingredients:

Avocado oil, for cooking

½ yellow onion, diced

1 garlic clove, minced

8.8 ounces (246 g) lean ground pork

2 tablespoons (28 ml) coconut aminos or tamari

1 teaspoon arrowroot powder

1 teaspoon grated fresh ginger

1 teaspoon ground ginger

½ teaspoon onion powder

½ teaspoon chile flakes

1 teaspoon salt

¼ teaspoon black pepper

½ cup shredded (35 g) green cabbage

½ cup shredded (35 g) red cabbage

½ cup (55 g) grated carrot

1 teaspoon sesame seeds

1 tablespoon (6 g) chopped green onion

Veggie Buddha Bowl

Featuring roasted vegetables, zucchini fritters, hard boiled eggs, and a drizzly tahini sauce, this Buddha bowl loaded with fiber and healthy fats for a filling and nutritious rest day meal.

Instructions:

1. Prepare the zucchini fritters ahead of time (see recipe on page 137). Preheat the oven to 350°F (180°C, or gas mark 4) and place the rack in the middle of the oven. Line a baking sheet with parchment paper.

2. Spread the asparagus, broccoli, and cauliflower on the prepared baking sheet. Sprinkle with paprika, ½ teaspoon of salt, and ¼ teaspoon of pepper and drizzle with a little olive oil. Toss to coat and then spread the vegetables out evenly on the sheet. Bake in oven for 20 to 25 minutes until the edges are golden.

3. While the vegetables are roasting, bring a large saucepan of water to a boil. Add the eggs and cook for 6 to 7 minutes until soft boiled. Remove from the heat, douse in cold water, peel, and set aside.

4. To prepare the salad, in a mixing bowl, combine the cucumber, tomato, carrot, salad greens, pepitas, coconut aminos, ½ teaspoon of salt, and ¼ teaspoon of pepper. Give everything a good toss to coat and set aside.

5. To make the tahini dip, combine all the ingredients in a small mixing bowl and vigorously stir until fully incorporated. It should form a loose dip. If the dip is too thick, add a touch more water until you reach the desired consistency.

6. Divide the salad between two bowls and top with the eggs, roasted vegetables, and zucchini fritters. Drizzle with the tahini dip, serve, and enjoy!

Difficulty: **Moderate**

Low Carb | High Protein | Vegetarian | Gluten Free | Grain Free | Dairy Free

Prep Time | 20 minutes

Cook Time | 25 minutes

Total Time | 45 minutes

Yield | 2 servings

Calories Per Serving | 288

Total Carbs | 10 g

Net Carbs | 6 g

Protein | 24 g

Fat | 18 g

Ingredients:

FOR THE BUDDHA BOWL:

6 zucchini fritters (see recipe on page 137)

6 asparagus spears, trimmed

1 cup (71 g) broccoli florets

1 cup (100 g) cauliflower florets

1 teaspoon smoked paprika

1 teaspoon salt

½ teaspoon black pepper

Olive oil, for cooking

4 large pasture-raised eggs

1 cucumber, diced

1 tomato, diced

½ carrot, grated

2 cups (110 g) mixed salad greens, washed

2 teaspoons pepitas

1 teaspoon coconut aminos or tamari

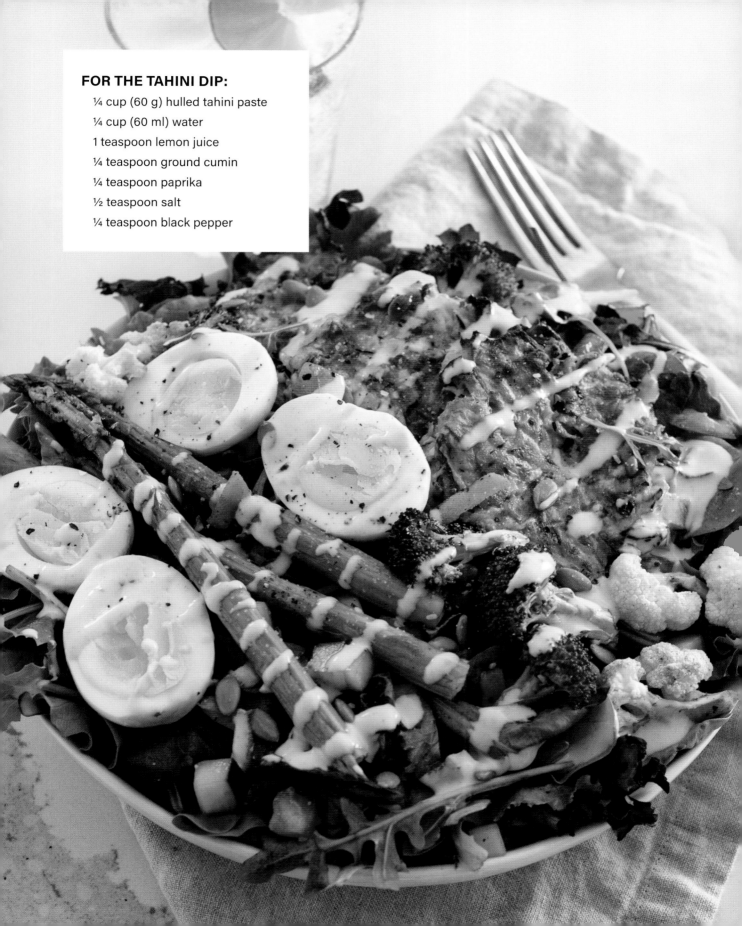

FOR THE TAHINI DIP:

¼ cup (60 g) hulled tahini paste

¼ cup (60 ml) water

1 teaspoon lemon juice

¼ teaspoon ground cumin

¼ teaspoon paprika

½ teaspoon salt

¼ teaspoon black pepper

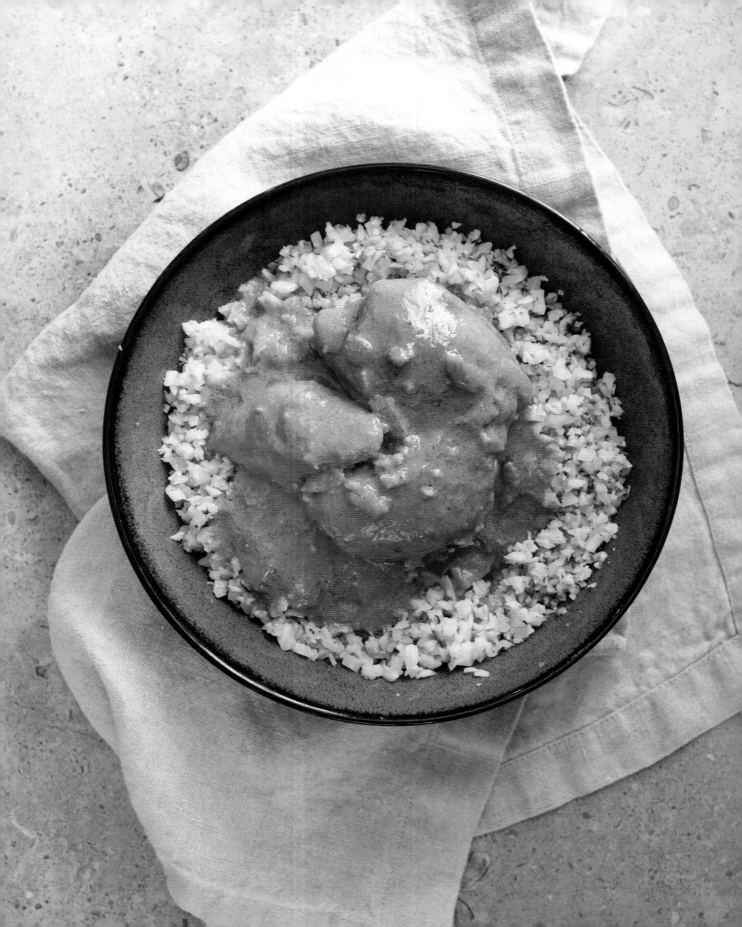

Butter Chicken with Cauliflower Rice

A healthy twist on a takeout favorite, this slow cooked chicken thigh dish in a creamy tomato sauce with traditional Indian spices is a nourishing high-protein meal.

Instructions:

1. Add a little coconut oil to a large skillet over medium-high heat or directly into your slow cooker pot if it has a sauté function. Once hot, add the onion, garlic, and ginger and cook until soft and fragrant, about 2 to 3 minutes. Add the garam masala, chili powder, curry powder, salt, pepper, and tomato paste and cook for another few minutes. If using a skillet, transfer the onions to the slow cooker pot at this point.

2. Place the chicken thighs on top of the mixture, pour the tomato purée over the chicken, and scatter the cubed butter over the top. Set the slow cooker on high for 2 to 3 hours or low for 4 to 6 hours until the chicken is cooked through and tender.

3. Just before serving, turn the slow cooker off and allow it to cool slightly. Add the coconut cream and yogurt and stir gently to combine.

4. To make the cauliflower rice, heat a little coconut oil in a large skillet over medium-high heat. Add the riced cauliflower and fry, stirring constantly until softened and tender, about 5 minutes.

5. Remove from the heat and divide the cauliflower rice between 6 serving bowls. Add a portion of the Butter Chicken on top and serve.

Notes

Please be aware that any ingredient additions, omissions, or substitutions will affect the nutritional information.

- For a dairy-free option, substitute coconut oil for the grass-fed butter and coconut cream for the Greek yogurt.
- Chicken thighs are ideal, but chicken breast, beef, or lamb can also be used.

Difficulty: **Easy**

Low Carb | High Protein | Gluten Free | Grain Free | Egg Free | Nut Free | Dairy Free (optional)

Prep Time | 15 minutes

Cook Time | 6 hours, 15 minutes

Total Time | 6 hours, 15 minutes

Yield | 6 servings

Calories Per Serving | 500

Total Carbs | 26 g

Net Carbs | 13 g

Protein | 38 g

Fat | 28 g

Ingredients:

Coconut oil, for cooking

1 yellow onion, diced

2 garlic cloves, minced

1 tablespoon (8 g) grated fresh ginger

1 tablespoon (7 g) garam masala powder

1 teaspoon chili powder

1 tablespoon (6 g) curry powder

1 teaspoon salt

¼ teaspoon black pepper

¾ cup (195 g) tomato paste

2 pounds (900 g) chicken thighs

1 can (14 ounces, or 390 g) tomato purée

2 tablespoons (28 g) grass-fed butter, cubed (see notes)

1 cup (244 g) full-fat coconut cream

1 cup (230 g) full-fat Greek yogurt (see notes)

6 cups (600 g) riced cauliflower

Turkey Stuffed Peppers

Since stuffed peppers are such a hit, we're featuring them again, this time minus the carb-heavy rice, but with the addition of vitamin B rich-turkey, to make it rest day-appropriate.

Instructions:

1. Preheat the oven to 375°F (190°C, or gas mark 5) and place the rack in the middle of the oven.

2. Place the bell peppers upside down in a large casserole dish, drizzle with olive oil, and season with a little salt and pepper. Roast in the oven for 15 to 20 minutes until softened and slightly browned. Remove from the heat and set aside.

3. While the peppers are baking, prepare the turkey filling. Add a little olive oil to a large skillet over medium heat. Add the yellow onion, green onion, and garlic and sauté until soft and translucent, about 3 to 5 minutes.

4. Add the ground turkey and cook for 5 minutes, breaking it up with a wooden spoon so that it browns evenly. Add the diced tomatoes (saving ¼ cup [60 ml] of the liquid for later), tomato purée, parsley, Italian seasoning, salt, and pepper. Stir to combine and cook for 5 minutes until the sauce thickens. Remove from the heat.

5. Arrange the bell peppers upright in the baking dish. Stuff the peppers by spooning the turkey mixture into the center cavity and top with the cheddar cheese.

6. Pour the reserved tomato liquid into the bottom of the dish and bake in the oven for 20 to 25 minutes or until the cheese is golden. Serve immediately while hot!

Notes

Please be aware that any ingredient additions, omissions, or substitutions will affect the nutritional information.

- Any lean ground meat works well in this recipe, such as chicken, pork, or beef.
- For a dairy-free option, omit the cheddar cheese.

Difficulty: **Moderate**

Low Carb | High Protein | Gluten Free | Grain Free | Dairy Free (optional) | Nut Free | Egg Free

Prep Time | 20 minutes

Cook Time | 25 minutes

Total Time | 45 minutes

Yield | 4 servings

Calories Per Serving | 299

Total Carbs | 14 g

Net Carbs | 10 g

Protein | 26 g

Fat | 15 g

Ingredients:

4 red bell peppers, tops, core, and seeds removed

Olive oil, for cooking

½ teaspoon salt, divided

¼ teaspoon black pepper, divided

⅓ cup (55 g) diced yellow onion

1 tablespoon (6 g) chopped green onion

1 garlic clove, minced

1 pound (455 g) ground turkey

1 can (14 ounces, or 390 g) diced tomatoes

½ cup (125 g) tomato purée

1 tablespoon (4 g) chopped fresh parsley

2 teaspoons Italian seasoning

¼ cup (30 g) shredded cheddar cheese (optional)

Sweet and Sour Beef

Skip the takeout! This homemade version of the popular Chinese dish is packed with protein, fresh bell peppers, and a zesty tomato sweet and sour sauce.

Instructions:

1. Heat a little avocado oil in a large wok or skillet over high heat. Add the onion and garlic and sauté for 2 to 3 minutes until soft and fragrant.

2. Add the beef strips and cook until browned on all sides, about 2 to 3 minutes. Lower the heat to medium and add the bell pepper. Cook for another 2 minutes, stirring occasionally, until softened.

3. Add the apple cider vinegar, tomato paste, coconut aminos, coconut sugar, and arrowroot powder. Stir well to combine.

4. Turn the heat back up to high and allow the liquid to simmer for a few minutes until it thickens. Remove from the heat and let sit for a few minutes before dividing into 4 serving bowls. Garnish with green onion and sesame seeds and serve.

Notes

Please be aware that any ingredient additions, omissions, or substitutions will affect the nutritional information.

- You can use any meat in this dish such as chicken or turkey.
- For a keto-friendly option, use erythritol or any low-carb sweetener in place of the coconut sugar.

Difficulty: **Moderate**

Low Carb | High Protein | Gluten Free | Grain Free | Dairy Free | Nut Free | Egg Free | Keto Friendly (optional)

Prep Time | 5 minutes

Cook Time | 15 minutes

Total Time | 20 minutes

Yield | 4 servings

Calories Per Serving | 345

Total Carbs | 15 g

Net Carbs | 13 g

Protein | 30 g

Fat | 18 g

Ingredients:

Avocado oil, for cooking

½ yellow onion, diced

1 garlic clove, minced

15 ounces (425 g) beef sirloin, cut into strips

1 red bell pepper, sliced

2 tablespoons (28 ml) apple cider vinegar

2 tablespoons (32 g) tomato paste

1 tablespoon (15 ml) coconut aminos or tamari

2 tablespoons (18 g) coconut sugar (see notes)

½ teaspoon arrowroot powder

1 tablespoon (6 g) chopped green onion

1 tablespoon (8 g) sesame seeds

Zucchini and Prosciutto "No Pasta" Lasagna

This "no pasta" lasagna is loaded with fiber-rich zucchini, salty prosciutto slices, and gooey mozzarella.

Instructions:

1. Preheat the oven to 350°F (180°C , or gas mark 4) and place the rack in the middle of the oven. Line a 9 x 5-inch (23 x 13-cm) loaf pan with parchment paper.

2. Mix the almond flour, Parmesan cheese, Italian seasoning, garlic powder, onion powder, paprika, salt, and pepper together in a small bowl and then transfer on to a small plate. In a separate small mixing bowl, beat the egg. Dip a zucchini strip in the egg mixture and then immediately dip into the flour mixture, turning the strip over so that the zucchini is fully coated. Transfer to a large plate and repeat for the remaining zucchini strips.

3. Sprinkle a tablespoon (15 ml) of the flour mixture on the bottom of the prepared pan. Add a layer of zucchini slices to the bottom of the pan, slightly overlapping each other. Add three slices of prosciutto on top, spoon 1 tablespoon (16 g) of tomato purée over the prosciutto, and top with ⅓ cup (38 g) of mozzarella cheese. Repeat the same steps for the next layer.

4. Top with a final layer of zucchini strips and sprinkle with the remaining mozzarella cheese and flour mixture. Transfer the pan to the oven and bake for 20 minutes. Then, turn the temperature up to 400°F (200°C, or gas mark 6) for the last 5 minutes until the top is golden brown and bubbly.

5. Remove from oven and let it cool for at least 10 minutes before serving.

Notes

The zucchinis are best sliced lengthwise using a vegetable peeler to create thin "ribbons." If you don't have a vegetable peeler, you can use a sharp knife, but try to slice them as thin as possible.

Difficulty: **Moderate**

Low Carb | High Protein | Gluten Free | Grain Free	
Prep Time | 5 minutes	
Cook Time | 25 minutes	
Total Time | 30 minutes	
Yield | 4 servings	
Calories Per Serving | 293	
Total Carbs | 9 g	
Net Carbs | 6 g	
Protein | 21 g	
Fat | 20 g	

Ingredients:

- ½ cup (56 g) almond flour
- ⅓ cup (33 g) grated Parmesan cheese
- 2 teaspoons Italian seasoning
- ½ teaspoon garlic powder
- ½ teaspoon onion powder
- ½ teaspoon paprika
- ¼ teaspoon salt
- ¼ teaspoon black pepper
- 1 large pasture-raised egg, beaten
- 2 medium zucchinis, thinly sliced (see notes)
- 6 thin slices prosciutto
- 2 tablespoons (31 g) tomato purée
- 1 cup (115 g) shredded mozzarella cheese
- Chile flakes (optional)

Pesto and Mozzarella Stuffed Chicken

A taste of Italy in under 20 minutes, this easy midweek dinner has all the nutrients you need for a break-day from the gym and features basil pesto, juicy sun-dried tomatoes, and gooey mozzarella cheese.

Instructions:

1. Make the pesto ahead of time. Add the pine nuts to a food processor and pulse a few times until coarse small pieces form (do not overprocess!). Add the remaining ingredients and pulse until the desired consistency is achieved. You may need to scrape down the sides a few times to ensure mixture is evenly processed.

2. Season both sides of each chicken breast with salt and pepper. Create a pocket for the filling in the center of each chicken breast by making a 3-inch (7.5 cm) cut through the side of each one, being careful not to slice all the way through. Stuff each breast with 1 tablespoon (15 g) of pesto, 2 tablespoons (15 g) of mozzarella cheese, and 4 sun-dried tomatoes. If needed, use a toothpick to hold the sides of the chicken breast together, securing the filling inside.

3. Heat a little olive oil in a large skillet over medium heat. Panfry each chicken breast until the cheese is melted and the chicken is golden brown and cooked through, about 6 to 8 minutes per side.

4. Transfer to a plate and serve with a side salad.

Notes

Please be aware that any ingredient additions, omissions, or substitutions will affect the nutritional information.

- Pesto can be stored in a mason jar in the fridge for up to a week.
- Any mild flavored oil, such as avocado or macadamia oil, works well in this pesto, but avoid unhealthy vegetable or seed oils. Macadamia nuts can also be substituted for the pine nuts in an equal measure.

Difficulty: **Easy**

High Protein	Low Carb	Gluten Free	Grain Free	
Prep Time	5 minutes	
Cook Time	20 minutes	
Total Time	25 minutes	
Yield	2 servings	
Calories Per Serving	517	
Total Carbs	7 g	
Net Carbs	2 g	
Protein	41 g	
Fat	42 g	

Ingredients:

FOR THE STUFFED CHICKEN:

- 2 large skinless boneless chicken breasts
- ¼ teaspoon salt
- ¼ teaspoon black pepper
- 2 tablespoons Basil and Pine Nut Pesto (recipe below)
- ¼ cup (30 g) shredded mozzarella cheese
- 8 sun-dried tomatoes or fresh cherry tomatoes, halved
- Olive oil, for cooking

FOR THE BASIL AND PINE NUT PESTO:

- ⅓ cup (45 g) pine nuts
- ⅓ cup (80 ml) olive oil
- 1 garlic clove
- 2 cups (48 g) fresh basil leaves
- ¼ teaspoon salt
- ¼ teaspoon black pepper
- ⅓ cup (33 g) grated Parmesan cheese (optional)

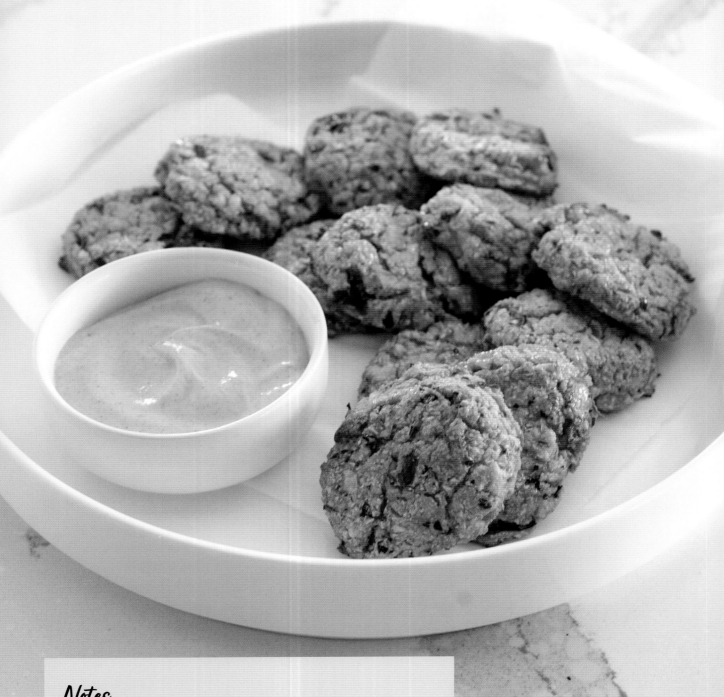

Notes

Make sure to use hulled tahini paste and not unhulled. Hulled tahini has had the outer shell removed from the seed and results in a milder flavor with the added benefit of higher absorption rates of calcium and other important minerals.

Cauliflower Falafel and Tahini Dip

A lighter take on the popular Middle Eastern staple, this falafel recipe uses cauliflower instead of chickpeas and the result is moist and flavorful. Whether you enjoy these as a midmorning snack or serve them at your next social gathering, once you try our delicious veggie-based falafel slathered in a creamy tahini dip, you won't go back!

Instructions:

1. Preheat the oven to 400°F (200°C, or gas mark 6) and place the rack in the middle of the oven. Line a baking sheet with parchment paper.

2. Add the cauliflower florets into a food processor and pulse until it forms a coarse rice-like texture. You may need to do this in two batches depending on the size of your food processor. Transfer the riced cauliflower into a large mixing bowl and set aside.

3. Add the parsley, onion, and garlic into the same food processor (no need to clean it out) and pulse until finely chopped. Transfer to the bowl with the cauliflower. Mix well to combine. Add the egg, almond flour, cumin, chili powder, turmeric, salt, and pepper and mix well to combine.

4. Using a cookie scoop, divide the mixture into 20 balls and place on the baking sheet. Bake for 35 to 40 minutes until golden brown and crispy, turning the baking sheet halfway through for even baking. Remove from the oven and let cool for a few minutes on a wire rack.

5. To make the tahini dip, combine all the ingredients in a small bowl and stir vigorously until fully incorporated. It should form a loose dip. If the dip is too thick, add a touch more water until you reach the desired consistency. If it's too loose, add a little more tahini paste.

6. Transfer the cauliflower falafel to a serving plate with the tahini dip and serve.

Difficulty: **Easy**

Low Carb | Vegetarian | Gluten Free | Grain Free

Prep Time | 10 minutes

Cook Time | 45 minutes

Total Time | 55 minutes

Yield | 4 servings (20 falafel)

Calories Per Serving | 177

Total Carbs | 10 g

Net Carbs | 7 g

Protein | 7 g

Fat | 13 g

Ingredients:

FOR THE CAULIFLOWER FALAFEL:

1 small cauliflower head, cut into florets

1 cup (60 g) chopped fresh parsley

½ small yellow onion

1 garlic clove

1 large pasture-raised egg

½ cup (56 g) almond flour

1 tablespoon (7 g) ground cumin

¼ teaspoon chili powder

½ teaspoon ground turmeric

1 teaspoon salt

½ teaspoon black pepper

FOR THE TAHINI DIP:

¼ cup (60 g) hulled tahini paste (see notes on page 150)

¼ cup (60 ml) water

1 teaspoon lemon juice

¼ teaspoon ground cumin

¼ teaspoon paprika

½ teaspoon salt

¼ teaspoon black pepper

Cheesy Bacon Fat Bomb

For all the bacon lovers out there, these fat "bombs" are a mouth-watering savory snack that combines aromatic dill, crunchy pickles, and cream cheese. It may sound indulgent, but it's actually full of healthy fats and protein to keep you full and nourished. What's not to love?

Instructions:

1. Heat a large skillet over medium-high heat. Add the bacon and cook until crispy, about 5 minutes per side. Remove from the heat and transfer to a paper towel-lined plate to absorb any excess fat.

2. Finely chop the bacon into bits and transfer to a small bowl. Add the green onion and mix to combine.

3. In a large mixing bowl, add the cream cheese, cheddar cheese, dill pickles, dill, and garlic powder and mix well to combine.

4. Using a cookie scoop or tablespoon, make 12 little balls out of the cream cheese mixture, rolling each ball in the bacon and green onion mixture to coat them fully. You may want to wash your hands between rolling each ball, as it will get quite messy!

5. Transfer to a serving plate and enjoy immediately.

Notes

Please be aware that any ingredient additions, omissions, or substitutions will affect the nutritional information.

For a vegetarian option, substitute sunflower seeds, pepitas, or sesame seeds for the chopped, cooked bacon.

Difficulty: **Easy**

Low Carb | High Protein | Gluten Free | Grain Free | Egg Free | Nut Free | Vegetarian (optional)

Prep Time | 15 minutes

Cook Time | 10 minutes

Total Time | 25 minutes

Yield | 6 servings (12 fat bombs)

Calories Per Serving | 164

Total Carbs | 2 g

Net Carbs | 2 g

Protein | 6 g

Fat | 15 g

Ingredients:

2 slices center-cut bacon (see notes)

1 green onion, finely chopped

1 cup (230 g) full-fat cream cheese

½ cup (58 g) shredded cheddar cheese

2 dill pickles, finely diced

1 tablespoon (4 g) chopped fresh dill

¼ teaspoon garlic powder

StrongCurves

Cottage Cheese and Avocado Bowl

Protein-packed cottage cheese, avocado slices, and juicy cherry tomatoes drizzled in hot sauce make this a simple yet delicious snack you can whip up in minutes.

Instructions:

1. Spoon the cottage cheese into a bowl and add the avocado and cherry tomatoes. Season with salt and pepper, drizzle with hot sauce, and serve.

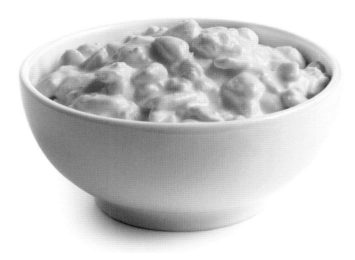

Low Carb | High Protein | Gluten Free | Grain Free | Egg Free | Nut Free | Vegetarian

Prep Time | 10 minutes

Total Time | 10 minutes

Yield | 1 serving

Calories Per Serving | 189

Total Carbs | 13 g

Net Carbs | 7 g

Protein | 14 g

Fat | 11 g

Ingredients:

1 cup (225 g) full-fat cottage cheese

½ large avocado, sliced

4 cherry tomatoes, halved

½ teaspoon salt

¼ teaspoon black pepper

Hot sauce, to drizzle (optional)

Spaghetti Squash Pizza Nests

Craving pizza but want a healthier low-carb option that's perfect for a recovery day snack? Packed with protein, these tasty little (gluten-free!) spaghetti squash nests are easy to make and feature the classic pizza combo of pepperoni and mozzarella cheese—though you can customize them with your own favorite toppings!

Instructions:

1. Preheat the oven to 400°F (200°C, or gas mark 6) and place the rack in the middle of the oven. Grease a muffin pan or line with silicone muffin liners.

2. Drizzle a little olive oil onto the flesh of each half of the squash. Rub the oil in with your fingertips to fully coat. Season with salt and pepper.

3. Place the squash on the baking sheet flesh-side down and pierce the skin a few times with a fork. Bake for 40 minutes or until golden on the outside and tender on the inside. You may need to bake for longer depending on the size of your squash, but do not overcook or the nests will turn mushy.

4. Remove from the oven and turn the squash halves over. Let cool for 5 minutes so they're easy to handle and then use a fork to scrape and fluff the strands from the sides of the squash. Using a cheesecloth or paper towels, squeeze as much excess liquid from the squash as possible before transferring it to a large mixing bowl.

5. Add the Parmesan cheese, eggs, and garlic powder and mix well to combine. Divide the mixture between the muffin cups and press each one down with spoon to create a well. Add a tablespoon (16 g) of tomato purée to each nest. Top with the mini pepperoni and shredded mozzarella cheese and garnish with the parsley.

6. Bake in the oven for 10 to 15 minutes until the nests are golden and the cheese is bubbly. Remove from the oven and let cool for a few minutes before serving.

Difficulty: **Easy**

Low Carb | High Protein | Gluten Free | Grain Free | Vegetarian (optional)

Prep Time | 10 minutes

Cook Time | 1 hour

Total Time | 1 hour, 10 minutes

Yield | 12 servings

Calories Per Serving | 117

Total Carbs | 7 g

Net Carbs | 6 g

Protein | 7 g

Fat | 7 g

Ingredients:

Olive oil, for baking

1 medium spaghetti squash, halved and seeds removed

Salt and black pepper, to taste

⅓ cup (33 g) grated Parmesan cheese

4 large pasture-raised eggs

1 teaspoon garlic powder

1½ cups (375 g) tomato purée

½ cup (69 g) mini pepperoni

1½ cups (175 g) shredded mozzarella cheese

1 tablespoon (4 g) chopped fresh parsley

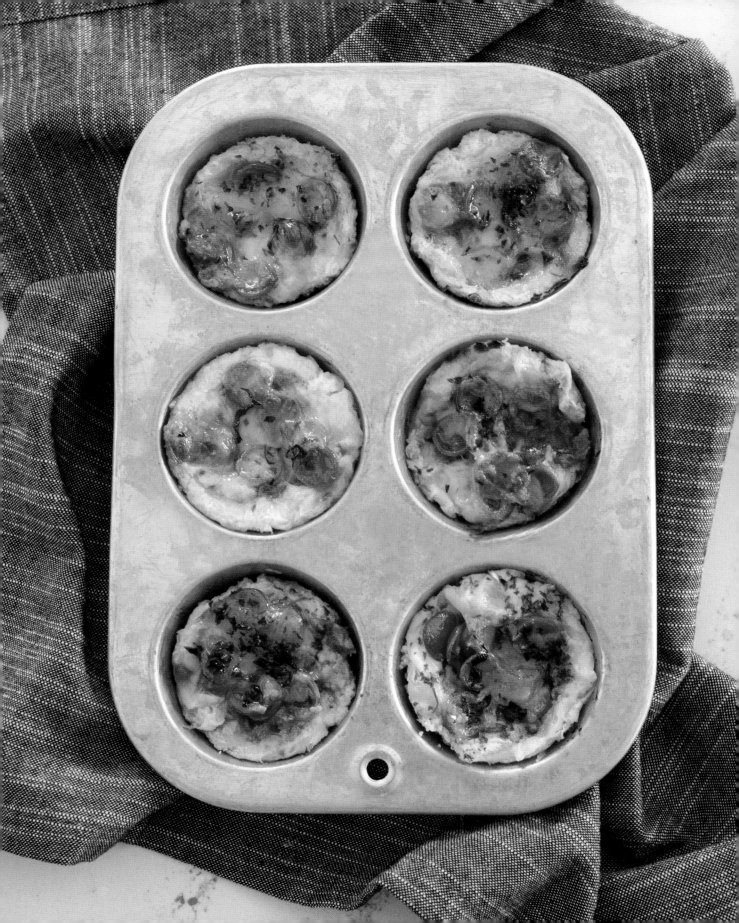

Nut Butter Buckeyes

High in fiber and healthy fats, yet low in sugar, these almond butter bites dipped in dark chocolate are a great treat to have on-hand when the sweet tooth hits in the afternoon—minus the sugar crash that comes after.

Instructions:

1. Line a baking sheet with parchment paper.

2. Melt the butter and almond butter in a small saucepan over low heat. Stir in the erythritol, vanilla, and salt until well-combined.

3. Remove the pan from the heat and add the almond flour. Mix with a spoon until a dough forms. Add more almond flour if the dough is slightly sticky.

4. Roll the dough into small truffle-sized balls (it makes about 24) and place on the baking sheet. Freeze for an hour until firm.

5. While the balls are in the freezer, prepare the chocolate coating. Add the chocolate and coconut oil to a heat-proof bowl over a small saucepan of simmering water on a low heat. Stir until fully melted.

6. Remove the chocolate from the heat and take the balls out of the freezer. Use a toothpick to skewer each ball and carefully roll in the melted chocolate.

7. Place back on the baking sheet and chill in the fridge for 30 minutes before serving.

Difficulty: **Easy**

Low Carb | Gluten Free | Grain Free | Egg Free | Vegetarian

Prep Time | 20 minutes | Chill: 30 minutes |Total: 50 minutes

Yield | 24 buckeyes

Calories Per Buckeye | 65

Total Carbs | 4 g

Net Carbs | 3 g

Protein | 1 g

Fat | 6 g

Ingredients:

5 tablespoons (70 g) grass-fed unsalted butter

¼ cup (65 g) almond butter

¼ cup (48 g) erythritol

1 teaspoon pure vanilla extract

½ teaspoon salt

½ cup (56 g) almond flour

3 ounces (85 g) 70–80% dark chocolate

½ tablespoon coconut oil

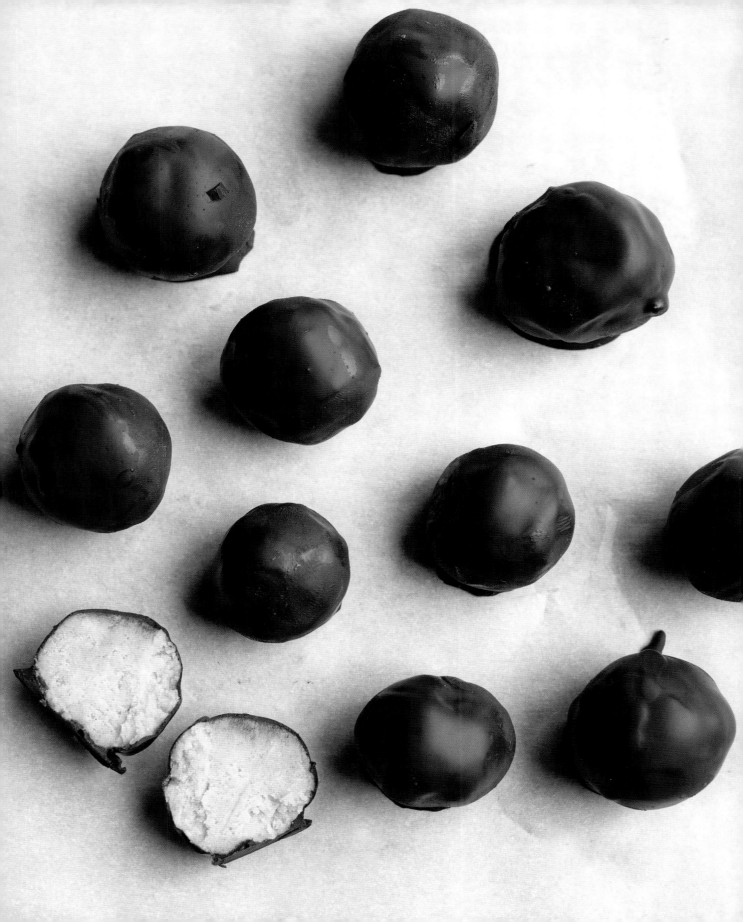

Crepes with Berries and Cream

These homemade crepes are making another appearance in this book—for good reason! They're a versatile and whole-food healthy base that you can use with so many toppings. This time, we're filling them with delicious sweet cream and mixed berries for a simple sweet treat that won't leave you nursing a sugar hangover for the rest of the day!

Instructions:

1. To make the crepe batter, add all the crepe ingredients to a food processor and pulse until fully incorporated and a loose batter forms.

2. Heat a little butter in a skillet over medium heat and ladle the batter in, swirling it around to evenly distribute. Cook until the top is firm, about 2 minutes. Flip and fry the other side until golden, another 2 to 3 minutes. Remove from the heat and let cool on a paper towel-lined plate.

3. Repeat with the remaining batter, wiping the pan clean after each time and using a little more butter as needed.

4. To assemble the crepe, spoon the whipped cream into the center, top with blueberries and strawberries, and serve immediately.

Notes

This recipe calls for psyllium husks, not psyllium husk powder. If using the latter, use half the amount shown in the recipe. Psyllium is a soluble fiber used in gluten-free baking for its binding properties and can be found in most health food stores and online.

Difficulty: **Moderate**

Low Carb | Vegetarian | Gluten Free | Grain Free

Prep Time | 5 minutes

Cook Time | 18 minutes

Total Time | 23 minutes

Yield | 1 crepe

Calories Per Serving | 179

Total Carbs | 10 g

Net Carbs | 7 g

Protein | 9 g

Fat | 14 g

Ingredients:

FOR THE CREPES (MAKES 6):

4 whole large pasture-raised eggs

4 large pasture-raised egg whites only

2 tablespoons (10 g) psyllium husk (see notes)

½ cup (115 g) full-fat cream cheese

Unsalted grass-fed butter, for frying

FOR THE FILLING:

1 tablespoon (15 ml) heavy cream, whipped

¼ cup (36 g) blueberries

¼ cup strawberries, halved

ANZAC Biscuits

This is a healthy twist on the patriotic Australian cookie commemorating the soldiers of the Australian and New Zealand Army Corps (ANZAC) during World War I. This golden, low-sugar, sliced almond cookie is perfectly soft and chewy.

Instructions:

1. Preheat the oven to 300°F (150°C, or gas mark 2) and place the rack in the middle of the oven. Line 2 baking sheets with parchment paper.

2. Combine the almond flour, sliced almonds, and desiccated coconut in a large mixing bowl. Set aside.

3. In a small saucepan over low heat, melt the butter, vanilla, and erythritol, stirring regularly. Simmer for 4 to 5 minutes until golden. Remove the pan from the heat and while still hot, stir in baking powder and water until fully combined. Add the wet ingredients to dry ingredients and stir until combined. Add the eggs to the mixture, beating well to incorporate. The dough will feel a little sticky, but don't worry! This means you'll end up with perfectly chewy cookies.

4. Using a tablespoon or cookie scoop, form the dough into roughly 16 balls and transfer to a cookie sheet. Using a thick-bottomed glass, flatten the balls into a cookie shape onto baking sheet, leaving 2 inches (5 cm) between each cookie.

5. Bake for 15 to 18 minutes until the edges are golden brown. Let cool on a rack for 5 minutes before serving.

Notes

Please be aware that any ingredient additions, omissions, or substitutions will affect the nutritional information.

- For a keto-friendly or low-carb option, any keto-friendly sweetener such as monk fruit or granulated stevia will work. If you prefer a natural sweetener, use coconut sugar instead of erythritol, but note that the carb count will be higher. Optionally, use half erythritol and half coconut sugar in equal measure for a low-sugar version.

Difficulty: **Easy**

Vegetarian | Strict Low Carb | Gluten Free | Grain Free | Keto Friendly (optional)

Prep Time | 10 minutes

Cook Time | 18 minutes

Total Time | 28 minutes

Yield | 16 cookies

Calories Per Cookie | 161

Total Carbs | 7 g

Net Carbs | 5 g

Protein | 5 g

Fat | 14 g

Ingredients:

1 cup (112 g) almond flour

1 cup (92 g) sliced almonds

1 cup (85 g) desiccated coconut

4 tablespoons (55 g) grass-fed butter

1 teaspoon pure vanilla extract

⅓ cup (64 g) erythritol (see notes)

1 teaspoon baking powder

1 teaspoon water

2 large pasture-raised eggs

Baklava Bites

These no-bake treats are inspired by the flavors of the popular Middle Eastern dessert baklava, but are super low in sugar and include good healthy fats from the pasture-fed butter and coconut as well as fiber from the nuts and seeds—a perfect rest day treat.

Instructions:

1. Line a baking sheet with parchment paper.

2. Add all the ingredients into a large mixing bowl and stir to combine.

3. Using a tablespoon or cookie scoop, form the mixture into small truffle-sized balls (it should make about 16) and place on the baking sheet. Chill and set in the fridge for 2 to 3 hours before serving.

Notes

You can use any mixed nuts of your choice, but pecans, walnuts, and pistachios work best for an authentic baklava flavor. Coarsely chopped nuts are ideal because they will keep their shape better as they chill in the fridge. You can also blend them coarsely in a food processor.

Difficulty: **Easy**

Low Carb | Gluten Free | Grain Free | Egg Free | Vegetarian

Prep Time | 20 minutes

Chill Time | 3 hours

Total Time | 3 hours, 20 minutes

Yield | 16 baklava bites

Calories Per Baklava Bite | 61

Total Carbs | 1 g

Net Carbs | 1 g

Protein | 2 g

Fat | 6 g

Ingredients:

¼ cup (55 g) grass-fed unsalted butter, melted

1 tablespoon (20 g) raw honey

1 teaspoon sesame seeds

1 tablespoon (9 g) sunflower seeds

1 tablespoon (9 g) pepitas

2 tablespoons (18 g) cup pine nuts

1 tablespoon (5 g) desiccated coconut

½ cup (73 g) mixed raw nuts, roughly chopped (see notes)

1 teaspoon ground cinnamon

¼ teaspoon salt

1 teaspoon pure vanilla extract

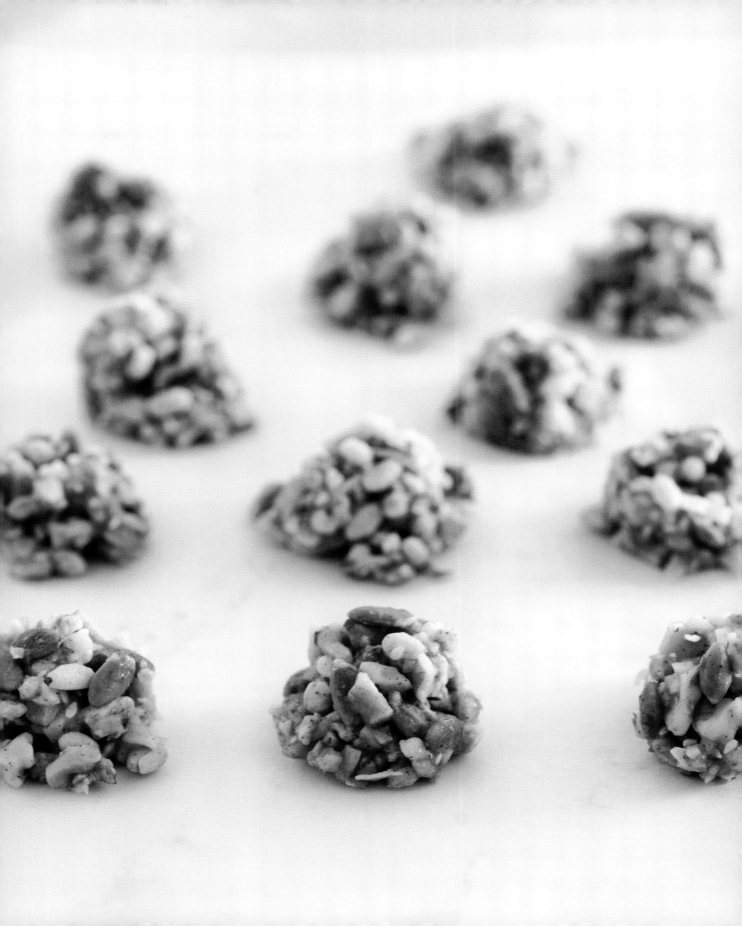

Peanut Butter Banana Muffins

Using only a few simple ingredients, these afternoon sweet treats are loaded with healthy fats and fiber, with a wonderful natural sweetness coming from the banana and honey. They're always a hit with the kids and a perfect snack while travelling too.

Instructions:

1. Preheat the oven to 350°F (180°C, or gas mark 4) and place the rack in the middle of the oven. Grease a muffin pan or line with silicone muffin liners.

2. Add the mashed bananas, eggs, honey, and vanilla extract to a large mixing bowl and whisk until combined. Add the almond flour, cinnamon, salt, and baking soda to the mixture and whisk until fully combined, making sure there are no lumps.

3. Spoon the banana batter into the muffin cups, filling each cup only halfway full. This should use up about half your batter.

4. Add a teaspoon of peanut butter directly on top of the batter in the center of each muffin and let it sink into the batter. If it doesn't sink in, help it along by pressing it down with the tip of the spoon.

5. Use the remaining batter to fill each muffin cup, distributing it evenly between the 12 cups and making sure the peanut butter is completely covered in each one.

6. Bake the muffins for 20 to 25 minutes until golden brown on the edges and a toothpick comes out clean. Transfer to a wire rack and let cool fully for at least 20 minutes before serving.

Notes

Please be aware that any ingredient additions, omissions, or substitutions will affect the nutritional information.

- It's best to use overripe bananas in this recipe as they add more sweetness and bake better than underripe bananas. The bananas should be a dark yellow color with plenty of dark spots and very soft on the inside.

- While this recipe is already low-carb, for those who are extra sensitive to carbs, simply use an equivalent amount of keto-friendly sweetener such as stevia, monk fruit, or erythritol in place of the honey.

Difficulty: **Easy**

Vegetarian | Low Carb | Gluten Free | Grain Free | Dairy Free

Prep Time | 10 minutes

Cook Time | 25 minutes

Total Time | 35 minutes

Yield | 12 muffins

Calories Per Muffin | 193

Total Carbs | 13 g

Net Carbs | 10 g

Protein | 7 g

Fat | 14 g

Ingredients:

2 large overripe bananas, mashed

3 large pasture-raised eggs

2 tablespoons (40 g) raw honey

1 tablespoon (15 ml) pure vanilla extract

2 cups (224 g) blanched and finely ground almond flour

1 tablespoon (7 g) ground cinnamon

¼ teaspoon Pink Himalayan or Celtic Sea Salt

1 teaspoon baking soda

4 tablespoons (65 g) natural peanut butter

Sugar-Free Hot Chocolate

This indulgent hot chocolate drink brings back comforting memories of warming your toes by the fire on a cold winter evening. It might taste like a dessert in a mug, but it's low in sugar and loaded with healthy fats from the milk and heavy cream.

Instructions:

1. Add the milk, erythritol, and raw cacao powder to a small saucepan over medium-low heat and whisk to combine.

2. Simmer on low for 3 to 4 minutes, whisking frequently, and then add the chocolate and salt. Continue to whisk until the chocolate has fully melted.

3. Pour into a mug, top with the whipped cream, and serve.

Notes

Please be aware that any ingredient additions, omissions, or substitutions will affect the nutritional information.

- For a dairy-free option, substitute unsweetened nut-free milk of your choice, such as coconut milk, for the full-fat cow's milk and substitute coconut cream for the heavy cream.

- This recipe is keto-friendly; however, if you prefer to use natural sugars instead of erythritol, use coconut sugar, raw honey, or 100% pure maple syrup to your taste.

- You can use other keto-friendly sweeteners such as monk fruit or stevia in place of erythritol too.

Difficulty: **Easy**

Low Carb | Sugar Free | Gluten Free | Grain Free | Egg Free | Nut Free | Dairy Free (optional) | Keto Friendly (optional)

Prep Time | 1 minute

Cook Time | 4 minutes

Total Time | 5 minutes

Yield | 1 serving

Calories Per Serving | 157

Total Carbs | 10 g

Net Carbs | 6 g

Protein | 3 g

Fat | 14 g

Ingredients:

1 cup (235 ml) full-fat cow's milk (see notes)

½ tablespoon erythritol, or more to taste (see notes)

1 tablespoon (5 g) raw cacao powder

1 square 70% dark chocolate (optional)

Pinch of salt

1 tablespoon (15 ml) heavy cream, whipped (optional)

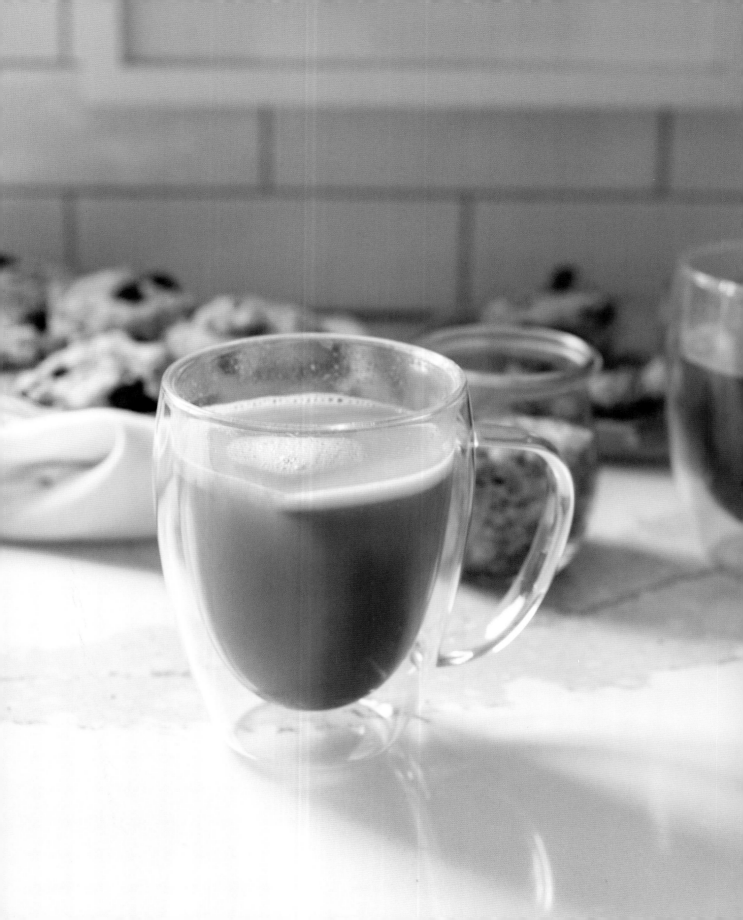

Sweet 'n Salty Fat Tea Latte

Curb your sweet tooth on your rest day with this indulgent, sweet, and creamy drink that tastes like dessert, but doesn't come with a massive sugar crash.

Instructions:

1. Prepare the tea in your favorite mug. Add the butter, salt, and stevia. Blend for a few seconds using a hand blender or whisk and enjoy!

Notes

Please be aware that any ingredient additions, omissions, or substitutions will affect the nutritional information.

For a dairy-free option, substitute the grass-fed butter with coconut oil or MCT oil.

Difficulty: **Easy**

Strict Low Carb | Sugar Free | Gluten Free | Grain Free | Egg Free | Nut Free | Dairy Free (optional)

Prep Time | 5 minutes

Total Time | 5 minutes

Yield | 1 serving

Calories Per Serving | 111

Total Carbs | 0 g

Net Carbs | 0 g

Protein | 0 g

Fat | 12 g

Ingredients:

1 cup (235 ml) strongly brewed hot tea of your choice, such as vanilla black tea

1 tablespoon (14 g) organic grass-fed butter or any healthy fat source of your choice (see notes)

Generous pinch of Himalayan pink rock salt

2–3 drops liquid stevia (or any low-carb sweetener of your choice)

Healing Bone Broth

Full of essential amino acids and collagen for optimal digestion, healthy skin, hair, and nails, drinking a cup or two (235 to 455 ml) of bone broth a day is a delicious and inexpensive way to enhance your health regime.

Instructions:

1. Add the chicken carcasses and feet or necks, carrots, onion, and any herbs or seasonings you may be using to a slow cooker or large stock pot. Fill the pot with cold water so that it covers the bones completely and add the apple cider vinegar. Let sit for 10 to 15 minutes to allow vinegar to pull the nutrients out of the bones.

2. Cover and cook on low for a minimum 24 hours. After 2 to 3 hours, remove any impurities floating in the top of your broth and discard.

3. Drain the liquid into a large bowl or several large mason jars and discard the bones and vegetables. Store broth in the fridge for up to a week. Once cooled, the fat will settle on the top, forming a crust. Either scrape it off and discard or reserve for cooking.

4. When ready to serve, reheat a cup (235 ml) of broth in a small saucepan over medium heat until it boils. Pour into a mug, season with a very generous pinch or up to ½ teaspoon of salt, and enjoy!

Notes

Please be aware that any ingredient additions, omissions, or substitutions will affect the nutritional information.

- Use any meat bones, fresh or frozen, but note that cooking times may vary depending on the bones used.
- Using chicken feet or necks is not essential, but the high amount of cartilage will give your broth a super gelatinous consistency for an extra collagen hit.
- You can customize this recipe using any herbs, spices, or vegetables you have on hand to your personal taste. However, it is best to add salt to taste once it's ready to serve.

Difficulty: **Easy**

Low Carb | High Protein | Gluten Free | Grain Free | Egg Free | Nut Free | Dairy Free

Prep Time | 5 minutes

Cook Time | 24 hours

Total Time | 24 hours, 5 minutes

Yield | 16 servings

Calories Per Serving | 37

Total Carbs | 1 g

Net Carbs | 1 g

Protein | 6 g

Fat | 1 g

Ingredients:

3–4 chicken carcasses

2 pounds (900 g) chicken feet or necks (optional)

2 carrots, chopped

1 yellow onion, chopped

Herbs and seasonings of your choice (optional)

3–7 gallons (5 to 7 L) filtered water

1 tablespoon (15 ml) apple cider vinegar

Pinch of salt, or more to taste, for serving

Adrenal Support Cocktail

This refreshing and fruity drink is loaded with vitamin C, magnesium, potassium, sodium, and essential amino acids to help support your cells, fight fatigue, and regulate your hormones. Whether you're feeling a little run-down or just need a pick me up after a stressful day, this adrenal cocktail has everything your body needs.

Instructions:

1. Combine all the ingredients in a large glass or jar and stir with a spoon.

Notes

Please be aware that any ingredient additions, omissions, or substitutions will affect the nutritional information.

- Pineapple juice also works well in this recipe, as long as it's 100% pure and fresh.
- Collagen is optional; however, it's an important component in this drink in order to balance blood sugar. As a substitute, use unflavored bone broth in equal parts to the other liquids. When choosing collagen powder, use a high-quality, clean collagen powder from grass-fed cows with no additives, fillers, gums, or anti-caking agents.

Difficulty: **Easy**

Low Carb | Sugar Free | Gluten Free | Grain Free | Egg Free | Nut Free | Dairy Free (optional)

Prep Time | 5 minutes

Total Time | 5 minutes

Yield | 2 servings

Calories Per Serving | 119

Total Carbs | 19 g

Net Carbs | 17 g

Protein | 11 g

Fat | 0 g

Ingredients:

1 cup (235 ml) 100% pure fresh orange juice

1 cup (235 ml) coconut water

½ teaspoon salt

2 scoops of unflavored collagen (optional)

Berry Collagen Shake

This light and fruity shake is made with sweet mixed berries, creamy almond butter, and an added boost of essential amino acids. It's also loaded with healthy fats from the almond butter, making this a delicious blood sugar-balancing drink on your rest days.

Instructions:

1. Combine all the ingredients in a blender and pulse for a few minutes until smooth and creamy.

2. Pour into a glass and serve immediately.

Notes

Please be aware that any ingredient additions, omissions, or substitutions will affect the nutritional information.

- Any nut butter will work in this recipe, such as cashew, peanut, or macadamia.

- Collagen is optional; however, it's an important component in this drink in order to balance blood sugar. As a substitute, use ½ cup (120 ml) of unflavored bone broth and ½ cup (120 ml) unsweetened almond milk. When choosing collagen powder, use a high-quality, clean collagen powder from grass-fed cows with no additives, fillers, gums, or anti-caking agents.

- You can sweeten this shake with a touch of raw honey or 100% pure maple syrup, to your taste.

Difficulty: **Easy**

Low Carb | Sugar Free | Gluten Free | Grain Free | Egg Free | Dairy Free (optional)

Prep Time | 5 minutes

Total Time | 5 minutes

Yield | 1 serving

Calories Per Serving | 238

Total Carbs | 21 g

Net Carbs | 18 g

Protein | 14 g

Fat | 12 g

Ingredients:

1 cup (235 ml) unsweetened almond milk

1 tablespoon (16 g) almond butter

½ cup (82 g) frozen mixed berries

½ teaspoon salt

1 scoop of unflavored collagen (optional)

StrongCurves

Notes

1. Austin, G. L., et al. (2009) A very low-carbohydrate diet improves symptoms and quality of life in diarrhea-predominant irritable bowel syndrome. Clin Gastroenterol Hepatol. 7(6):706–708.e1.

2. Bauer J., et al. (2013) Evidence-based recommendations for optimal dietary protein intake in older people: a position paper from the PROT-AGE Study Group. J Am Med Dir Assoc. 14(8):542–59.

3. Carroll, P. V., et al. (1998) Growth hormone deficiency in adulthood and the effects of growth hormone replacement: a review. Growth Hormone Research Society Scientific Committee. J Clin Endocrinol Metab. 83(2):382–395.

4. Chavarro, J. E., et al. (2007) A prospective study of dairy foods intake and anovulatory infertility. Hum Reprod. 22(5):1340–7.

5. Corkey B. E. (2012) Banting lecture 2011: hyperinsulinemia: cause or consequence? Diabetes. 61(1):4–13.

6. Covassin, N., et al. (2016) Keeping up with the clock: circadian disruption and obesity risk. Hypertension. 68(5):1081–1090.

7. Davidson, J. R., et al. (1991) Growth hormone and cortisol secretion in relation to sleep and wakefulness. J Psychiatry Neurosci. 16(2):96–102.

8. DiNicolantonio, J. J. and O'Keefe, J. H. (2018) Omega-6 vegetable oils as a driver of coronary heart disease: the oxidized linoleic acid hypothesis. Open Heart. 5(2):e000898.

9. Gibson, A. A., et al. (2015) Do ketogenic diets really suppress appetite? A systematic review and meta-analysis. Obes Rev. 16(1):64–76.

10. Helge, J. W. (2017) A high carbohydrate diet remains the evidence based choice for elite athletes to optimise performance. J Physiol. 595(9):2775.

11. Hernandez, A. R., et al. (2018) A ketogenic diet improves cognition and has biochemical effects in prefrontal cortex that are dissociable from hippocampus. Front Aging Neurosci. 10:391.

12. Kniskern, M. A., et al. (2011) Protein dietary reference intakes may be inadequate for vegetarians if low amounts of animal protein are consumed. Nutrition. 27(6):727–30.

13. Layman, D. K., et al. (2015) Defining meal requirements for protein to optimize metabolic roles of amino acids. Am J Clin Nutr. 101(6):1330S-1338S.

14. Layman, D. K. (2009) Dietary Guidelines should reflect new understandings about adult protein needs. Nutr Metab. 6:12.

15. Martin, C. K., et al. (2011) Change in food cravings, food preferences, and appetite during a low-carbohydrate and low-fat diet. Obesity (Silver Spring). 19(10):1963-1970.

16. Mozaffarian, D. (2016) Dietary fat. In: Encyclopedia of Food and Health, vol. 2, pp. 163–170.

17. Nair, K. S., et al. (1988) Effect of beta-hydroxybutyrate on whole-body leucine kinetics and fractional mixed skeletal muscle protein synthesis in humans. J Clin Invest. 82(1):198–205.

18. Noakes, M., et al. (2006) Comparison of isocaloric very low carbohydrate/high saturated fat and high carbohydrate/low saturated fat diets on body composition and cardiovascular risk. Nutr Metab (Lond). 3:7.

19. Nuttall, F. Q., et al. (2015) Comparison of a carbohydrate-free diet vs. fasting on plasma glucose, insulin and glucagon in type 2 diabetes. Metabolism. 64(2):253-62.

20. Nuttall, F. Q., et al. (2016) The ghrelin and leptin responses to short-term starvation vs a carbohydrate-free diet in men with type 2 diabetes; a controlled, cross-over design study. Nutr Metab (Lond). 13:47.

21. Pasiakos, S. M., et al. (2013) Effects of high-protein diets on fat-free mass and muscle protein synthesis following weight loss: a randomized controlled trial. FASEB J. 27(9):3837–3847.

22. Patel, H., et al. (2017) Aerobic vs anaerobic exercise training effects on the cardiovascular system. World J Cardiol. 9(2):134–138.

23. Ramsden, C. E., et al. (2010) n-6 fatty acid-specific and mixed polyunsaturate dietary interventions have different effects on CHD risk: a meta-analysis of randomised controlled trials. Br J Nutr. 104(11):586–600.

24. Rogerson, D. (2017) Vegan diets: practical advice for athletes and exercisers. J Int Soc Sports Nutr. 14:36.

Acknowledgments

25. Rutherfurd, S. M., et al. (2015) Protein digestibility-corrected amino acid scores and digestible indispensable amino acid scores differentially describe protein quality in growing male rats. J Nutr. 145(2):372–9.

26. Sainsbury, E., et al. (2018) Effect of dietary carbohydrate restriction on glycemic control in adults with diabetes: A systematic review and meta-analysis. Diabetes Res Clin Pract. 139:239–252.

27. Saslow, L. R., et al. (2017) Twelve-month outcomes of a randomized trial of a moderate-carbohydrate versus very low-carbohydrate diet in overweight adults with type 2 diabetes mellitus or prediabetes. Nutr Diabetes. 7(12):304.

28. Smith, R. N., et al. (2007) The effect of a high-protein, low glycemic-load diet versus a conventional, high glycemic-load diet on biochemical parameters associated with acne vulgaris: a randomized, investigator-masked, controlled trial. J Am Acad Dermatol. 57(2):247–56.

29. Takahashi, Y., et al. (1968) Growth hormone secretion during sleep. J Clin Invest. 47(9):2079–2090.

30. Tarnopolsky, M. A. (2008) Sex differences in exercise metabolism and the role of 17-beta estradiol. Med Sci Sports Exerc. 40(4):648–54.

31. Templeman N. M., et al. (2017) A causal role for hyperinsulinemia in obesity. J Endocrinol. 232(3):R173–R183.

32. Trexler, E. T., et al. (2014) Effects of dietary macronutrient distribution on resting and post-exercise metabolism. J Int Soc Sports Nutr. 11(1):P6.

33. Watson, A. M. (2017) Sleep and athletic performance. Curr Sports Med Rep. 16(6):413–418.

34. Weigle, D. S., et al. (2005) A high-protein diet induces sustained reductions in appetite, ad libitum caloric intake, and body weight despite compensatory changes in diurnal plasma leptin and ghrelin concentrations. Am J Clin Nutr. 82(1):41–8.

35. Westman, E. C. (2002) Is dietary carbohydrate essential for human nutrition? Am J Clin Nutr. 75(5):951–953.

36. Wilcox G. (2005) Insulin and insulin resistance. Clin Biochem. 26(2):19–39.

37. Wu G. (2016) Dietary protein intake and human health. Food Funct. 7(3):1251–65.

Writing this cookbook has been an incredible journey, and I am so grateful to everyone who has supported me along the way. First and foremost, I want to thank my partner (and Chief Recipe Taster!), Adam, who has always encouraged me to pursue my passions and believed in me, even when I have doubted myself. Without his love and unwavering support, none of this would have been possible.

I am also grateful to the team at Fair Winds and Quarto. With a special mention for my editor, Hilary, who has worked diligently to bring this cookbook to life. With your guidance and invaluable expertise, working on my first book has been a joy and I could not be more proud of the end result. Thank you for believing in me and making this lifelong dream of mine a reality.

To all of the incredible women who have shared their fitness journeys with me over the years, whether in person, through my Strong Curves app or YouTube channel, thank you for inspiring me and motivating me to keep pushing forward. I wouldn't be where I am today, if it wasn't for you.

Finally, I want to thank the readers of this cookbook. Whether you are a seasoned athlete or a newcomer to the world of fitness and nutrition, I hope that these recipes will inspire you to take control of your health and achieve your goals. Thank you for trusting me and allowing me to be a part of your journey towards a stronger, healthier you.

About the Author

Shelley Darlington is the founder of Strong Curves, a brand that empowers women to become the master of their body, without gimmicks or deprivation. With the Strong Curves app, her digital guides, fitness equipment, and now, cookbook, Shelley offers every resource a woman could need on her health and fitness journey.

Shelley is a certified personal trainer, yoga teacher, nutritionist, and health and wellness coach, with over a decade of experience in the fitness industry. Currently living in Australia, she says her recipes are inspired by her multicultural upbringing and love of travel. She is an advocate for animal-based nutrition, and her creative process involves reimagining comfort foods and popular dishes and turning them into healthier versions using nutrient-dense, whole foods.

Shelley strongly believes that fitness and nutrition go hand in hand and that a healthy diet is the foundation of any fitness program. Through Strong Curves, Shelley has helped thousands of women from all over the world to build strength, gain confidence, and improve their health. Her no-fuss approach is grounded in science and practicality, and she truly believes that anyone can achieve their fitness goals with the right mindset, knowledge, and support.

You can find more healthy recipes, workouts and fitness tips on her website www.shelleydarlington.com and join her fast growing Strong Curves app at www.strongcurvesapp.com.

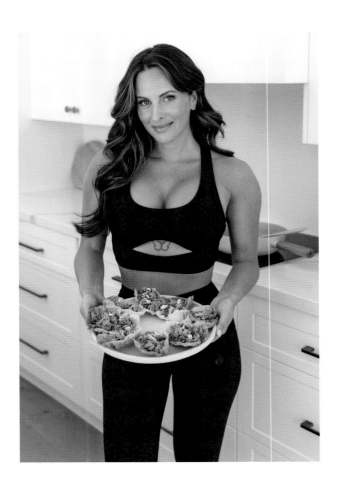

Index

A

almond butter
Almond Butter and Banana Rice Cakes, 102
Berry Collagen Shake, 168
Coconut Energy Balls, 118
No-Bake Protein Bar, 103
Nut Butter Buckeyes, 156
Protein Brownies, 117
almond milk
Berry Collagen Shake, 168
Cherry Chocolate Masa Bowl, 75
Chocolate Mint Smoothie Bowl, 30
No-Bake Protein Bar, 103
Peanut Butter Banana Smoothie, 111
Vanilla Protein Pudding, 37
almonds: ANZAC Biscuits, 159
apples: Cinnamon Apple with Nut Butter, 104
apricots: Apricot Breakfast Bake, 72
asparagus: Veggie Buddha Bowl, 142–143
avocados
Avo Egg Smash, 127
BLT Pasta Salad, 86
Chicken and Avocado Lettuce Wraps, 42
Chocolate Mint Smoothie Bowl, 30
Cottage Cheese and Avocado Bowl, 153
Cottage Cheese and Avocado Rice Cakes, 102
Green Goddess Smoothie, 112
Salmon and Cream Cheese Sushi, 128
Shrimp-Stuffed Avocado, 132
Sweet Potato Avocado Boats, 101
Zesty Salmon Power Bowl, 33

B

bacon
BLT Pasta Salad, 86
Cheesy Bacon Fat Bomb, 152
Egg Salad Wrap, 43
Fuel-Up Breakfast Burger, 36
Full English Breakfast Quesadilla, 34
Mushroom and Bacon Soup, 135
bananas
Almond Butter and Banana Rice Cakes, 102
Banana Protein Pancakes, 74
Chocolate Malt Collagen Shake, 116
Chocolate Mint Smoothie Bowl, 30
Peanut Butter Banana Muffins, 162
Peanut Butter Banana Smoothie, 111
Strawberry Oatmeal Smoothie, 114
beans, black: Taco Nachos with Salsa, 88–89
beans, green
Sautéed Green Beans and Mushrooms, 65
Warm Steak Salad, 40
beans, kidney: Chili Con Carne, 95

beef
Beef and Rice Stuffed Peppers, 98
Chili Con Carne, 95
Stuffed Cabbage Rolls, 52
Sweet and Sour Beef, 147
Taco Nachos with Salsa, 88–89
Warm Steak Salad, 40
bell peppers
Beef and Rice Stuffed Peppers, 98
Chicken Enchiladas, 90–91
Chili Con Carne, 95
Mexican-Style Egg Frittata, 32
One Pan Moroccan Potato Hash, 97
Red Thai Curry with Shrimp, 92
Sweet and Sour Beef, 147
Turkey Stuffed Peppers, 146
berries, mixed
Berry Collagen Shake, 168
Frozen Yogurt Bites, 123
Grain-Free Granola, 130
Greek Yogurt and Berries, 58
Vanilla Protein Pudding, 37
blueberries
Blueberry and Zucchini Muffins, 60
Blueberry Breakfast Bake, 131
Crepes with Berries and Cream, 158
Grain-Free Porridge, 126
Greek Yogurt and Berries, 58
bok choy: Teriyaki Salmon and Bok Choy, 44
broccoli
Cheesy Broccoli Poppers, 66
Mini Salmon Broccoli Quiche, 138
Veggie Buddha Bowl, 142–143

C

cabbage
Crispy Shrimp Rice Paper Rolls, 85
Pork Egg Roll in a Bowl, 141
Pork San Choi Bao, 39
Red Cabbage Slaw, 64
Stuffed Cabbage Rolls, 52
Sweet Potato and Turkey Quinoa Bowl, 81
carrots
Crispy Shrimp Rice Paper Rolls, 85
Healing Bone Broth, 166
Pork Egg Roll in a Bowl, 141
Pork San Choi Bao, 39
Red Cabbage Slaw, 64
Veggie Buddha Bowl, 142–143
cashew butter
Chocolate Malt Collagen Shake, 116
Honey Puffed Rice Bars, 120
cashews: Pork San Choi Bao, 39
cauliflower
Butter Chicken with Cauliflower Rice, 145
Cauliflower Falafel and Tahini Dip, 151
Chicken and Sweet Corn Soup, 46
Stuffed Cabbage Rolls, 52
Veggie Buddha Bowl, 142–143

cheddar cheese
    Beef and Rice Stuffed Peppers, 98
    Cheesy Bacon Fat Bomb, 152
    Cheesy Broccoli Poppers, 66
    Cheesy Chicken Patties, 139
    Chicken Enchiladas, 90–91
    Full English Breakfast Quesadilla, 34
    Ham and Egg Cups, 41
    Hummus, Turkey, and Cheese Rice Cakes, 102
    Stuffed Cabbage Rolls, 52
    Taco Nachos with Salsa, 88–89
    Turkey Stuffed Peppers, 146
cherries: Cherry Chocolate Masa Bowl, 75
chicken
    Butter Chicken with Cauliflower Rice, 145
    Cheesy Chicken Patties, 139
    Chicken and Avocado Lettuce Wraps, 42
    Chicken and Sweet Corn Soup, 46
    Chicken Enchiladas, 90–91
    Chicken Shish Taouk Skewers, 50
    Creamy Tuscan Chicken, 49
    Healing Bone Broth, 166
    Italian Meatballs, 47
    Pesto and Mozzarella Stuffed Chicken, 149
chickpeas: Stuffed Mushrooms, 69
chocolate
    Cherry Chocolate Masa Bowl, 75
    Chewy Fig Protein Bar, 62
    Chocolate Malt Collagen Shake, 116
    Chocolate Mint Smoothie Bowl, 30
    No-Bake Protein Bar, 103
    Nut Butter Buckeyes, 156
    Protein Brownies, 117
    Protein-Packed Chocolate Pudding, 121
    Sugar-Free Hot Chocolate, 163
coconut
    ANZAC Biscuits, 159
    Baklava Bites, 160
    Chewy Fig Protein Bar, 62
    Chocolate Mint Smoothie Bowl, 30
    Coconut Energy Balls, 118
coconut cream: Butter Chicken with Cauliflower Rice, 145
coconut flour: Blueberry Breakfast Bake, 131
coconut milk
    Creamy Tuscan Chicken, 49
    Red Thai Curry with Shrimp, 92
coconut sugar
    Apricot Breakfast Bake, 72
    Blueberry and Zucchini Muffins, 60
    Chewy Fig Protein Bar, 62
    Protein Brownies, 117
    Red Thai Curry with Shrimp, 92
coconut water
    Adrenal Support Cocktail, 167
    Electrolyte Replenisher, 115
corn
    Chicken and Sweet Corn Soup, 46
    Red Thai Curry with Shrimp, 92

    Tuna and Mayo Topped Baked Potato, 87
cottage cheese
    Cottage Cheese and Avocado Bowl, 153
    Cottage Cheese and Avocado Rice Cakes, 102
    Protein-Packed Chocolate Pudding, 121
cream cheese
    Cheesy Bacon Fat Bomb, 152
    Crepes with Berries and Cream, 158
    Salmon and Cream Cheese Crepes, 136
    Salmon and Cream Cheese Sushi, 128
    Salmon and Cucumber Canapés, 57
    Salmon Sushi Bake, 94
cucumber
    Chop-Chop Salad, 63
    Green Goddess Smoothie, 112
    Protein Bento Box, 59
    Salmon and Cream Cheese Sushi, 128
    Salmon and Cucumber Canapés, 57
    Veggie Buddha Bowl, 142–143
    Warm Steak Salad, 40
    Zesty Salmon Power Bowl, 33

D

dates
    Chocolate Malt Collagen Shake, 116
    Coconut Energy Balls, 118

E

eggs
    ANZAC Biscuits, 159
    Apricot Breakfast Bake, 72
    Avo Egg Smash, 127
    Baked Spinach and Feta Tortilla, 140
    Banana Protein Pancakes, 74
    BLT Pasta Salad, 86
    Blueberry and Zucchini Muffins, 60
    Cauliflower Falafel and Tahini Dip, 151
    Cheesy Broccoli Poppers, 66
    Cheesy Chicken Patties, 139
    Cherry Chocolate Masa Bowl, 75
    Chicken and Sweet Corn Soup, 46
    Crepes with Berries and Cream, 158
    Egg and Feta Muffins, 129
    Egg Salad Wrap, 43
    Fuel-Up Breakfast Burger, 36
    Full English Breakfast Quesadilla, 34
    Grain-Free Granola, 130
    Ham and Egg Cups, 41
    Herbed Latkes, 106
    Japanese-Style Egg and Rice, 79
    Mexican-Style Egg Frittata, 32
    Mini Salmon Broccoli Quiche, 138
    New York Deli Breakfast Burrito, 76
    One Pan Moroccan Potato Hash, 97
    Peanut Butter Banana Muffins, 162

Pesto Deviled Eggs, 105
Protein Bento Box, 59
Salmon and Cream Cheese Crepes, 136
Savory Oatmeal with a Poached Egg, 80
Shakshuka (Eggs Poached in Tomato Sauce), 82
Spaghetti Squash Pizza Nests, 154
Veggie Buddha Bowl, 142–143
Zucchini and Prosciutto "No Pasta" Lasagna, 148
Zucchini Fritters with Fried Eggs, 137

F

feta cheese
    Baked Spinach and Feta Tortilla, 140
    Egg and Feta Muffins, 129
    Protein Bento Box, 59
figs: Chewy Fig Protein Bar, 62

G

garlic
    Beef and Rice Stuffed Peppers, 98
    Butter Chicken with Cauliflower Rice, 145
    Cauliflower Falafel and Tahini Dip, 151
    Cheesy Broccoli Poppers, 66
    Cheesy Chicken Patties, 139
    Chicken and Sweet Corn Soup, 46
    Chicken Enchiladas, 90–91
    Chicken Shish Taouk Skewers, 50
    Chili Con Carne, 95
    Creamy Tuscan Chicken, 49
    Crispy Shrimp Rice Paper Rolls, 85
    Grilled Shrimp and Zucchini Salad, 54
    Italian Meatballs, 47
    Mushroom and Bacon Soup, 135
    Mushroom Pearl Couscous, 108
    New York Deli Breakfast Burrito, 76
    One Pan Moroccan Potato Hash, 97
    Pesto and Mozzarella Stuffed Chicken, 149
    Pesto Deviled Eggs, 105
    Pork Egg Roll in a Bowl, 141
    Pork San Choi Bao, 39
    Red Thai Curry with Shrimp, 92
    Sautéed Green Beans and Mushrooms, 65
    Savory Oatmeal with a Poached Egg, 80
    Shakshuka (Eggs Poached in Tomato Sauce), 82
    Stuffed Cabbage Rolls, 52
    Stuffed Mushrooms, 69
    Sweet and Sour Beef, 147
    Teriyaki Salmon and Bok Choy, 44
    Turkey Stuffed Peppers, 146
    Warm Steak Salad, 40
greens
    Grilled Shrimp and Zucchini Salad, 54
    Sweet Potato and Turkey Quinoa Bowl, 81
    Veggie Buddha Bowl, 142–143
Gruyère cheese: Tuna Casserole, 53

H

ham: Ham and Egg Cups, 41
hummus
    Hummus, Turkey, and Cheese Rice Cakes, 102
    Protein Bento Box, 59

J

jalapeños: Taco Nachos with Salsa, 88–89

K

kiwi: Green Goddess Smoothie, 112

L

lemongrass: Red Thai Curry with Shrimp, 92
lettuce
    BLT Pasta Salad, 86
    Chicken and Avocado Lettuce Wraps, 42
    Fuel-Up Breakfast Burger, 36
    Pork San Choi Bao, 39

M

mozzarella cheese
    Baked Spinach and Feta Tortilla, 140
    Pesto and Mozzarella Stuffed Chicken, 149
    Spaghetti Squash Pizza Nests, 154
    Zucchini and Prosciutto "No Pasta" Lasagna, 148
mushrooms
    Chicken Enchiladas, 90–91
    Crispy Shrimp Rice Paper Rolls, 85
    Mexican-Style Egg Frittata, 32
    Mushroom and Bacon Soup, 135
    Mushroom Pearl Couscous, 108
    Sautéed Green Beans and Mushrooms, 65
    Stuffed Mushrooms, 69
    Warm Steak Salad, 40

N

nuts, mixed
    Baklava Bites, 160
    Chewy Fig Protein Bar, 62
    Grain-Free Granola, 130

O

oats
    Apricot Breakfast Bake, 72
    Banana Protein Pancakes, 74
    No-Bake Protein Bar, 103
    Savory Oatmeal with a Poached Egg, 80
    Strawberry Oatmeal Smoothie, 114
olives: Protein Bento Box, 59
onions
    Baked Spinach and Feta Tortilla, 140
    Beef and Rice Stuffed Peppers, 98
    BLT Pasta Salad, 86
    Butter Chicken with Cauliflower Rice, 145

Cauliflower Falafel and Tahini Dip, 151
Cheesy Bacon Fat Bomb, 152
Chicken and Avocado Lettuce Wraps, 42
Chicken and Sweet Corn Soup, 46
Chicken Enchiladas, 90–91
Chili Con Carne, 95
Creamy Tuscan Chicken, 49
Crispy Shrimp Rice Paper Rolls, 85
Fuel-Up Breakfast Burger, 36
Grilled Shrimp and Zucchini Salad, 54
Ham and Egg Cups, 41
Healing Bone Broth, 166
Herbed Latkes, 106
Japanese-Style Egg and Rice, 79
Mexican-Style Egg Frittata, 32
Mushroom and Bacon Soup, 135
Mushroom Pearl Couscous, 108
New York Deli Breakfast Burrito, 76
One Pan Moroccan Potato Hash, 97
Pork Egg Roll in a Bowl, 141
Pork San Choi Bao, 39
Salmon Sushi Bake, 94
Shakshuka (Eggs Poached in Tomato Sauce), 82
Stuffed Cabbage Rolls, 52
Stuffed Mushrooms, 69
Sweet and Sour Beef, 147
Taco Nachos with Salsa, 88–89
Tuna Casserole, 53
Turkey Stuffed Peppers, 146
Zesty Salmon Power Bowl, 33
orange juice
    Adrenal Support Cocktail, 167
    Chewy Fig Protein Bar, 62

P

Parmesan cheese
    Pesto and Mozzarella Stuffed Chicken, 149
    Pesto Deviled Eggs, 105
    Spaghetti Squash Pizza Nests, 154
    Stuffed Mushrooms, 69
    Zucchini and Prosciutto "No Pasta" Lasagna, 148
pasta: BLT Pasta Salad, 86
pastrami
    New York Deli Breakfast Burrito, 76
    Sweet Potato Avocado Boats, 101
peanut butter
    Cinnamon Apple with Nut Butter, 104
    Peanut Butter Banana Muffins, 162
    Peanut Butter Banana Smoothie, 111
pears: Green Goddess Smoothie, 112
peas, snow: Red Thai Curry with Shrimp, 92
pecans: Blueberry Breakfast Bake, 131
pepitas
    Baklava Bites, 160
    Grain-Free Granola, 130
    Red Cabbage Slaw, 64
    Sweet Potato and Turkey Quinoa Bowl, 81
    Veggie Buddha Bowl, 142–143

pepperoni: Spaghetti Squash Pizza Nests, 154
pickles
    Cheesy Bacon Fat Bomb, 152
    Egg Salad Wrap, 43
    Fuel-Up Breakfast Burger, 36
    New York Deli Breakfast Burrito, 76
pine nuts
    Baklava Bites, 160
    Pesto and Mozzarella Stuffed Chicken, 149
    Pesto Deviled Eggs, 105
    Sautéed Green Beans and Mushrooms, 65
    Warm Steak Salad, 40
pork
    Italian Meatballs, 47
    Pork Egg Roll in a Bowl, 141
    Pork San Choi Bao, 39
potatoes
    Herbed Latkes, 106
    New York Deli Breakfast Burrito, 76
    Tuna and Mayo Topped Baked Potato, 87
prosciutto: Zucchini and Prosciutto "No Pasta" Lasagna, 148

Q

quinoa
    Peanut Butter Banana Smoothie, 111
    Sweet Potato and Turkey Quinoa Bowl, 81
    Zesty Salmon Power Bowl, 33

R

raisins: Apricot Breakfast Bake, 72
raspberries: Greek Yogurt and Berries, 58
rice
    Beef and Rice Stuffed Peppers, 98
    Bone Broth Rice, 110
    Butter Chicken with Cauliflower Rice, 145
    Chili Con Carne, 95
    Honey Puffed Rice Bars, 120
    Japanese-Style Egg and Rice, 79
    Red Thai Curry with Shrimp, 92
    Salmon Sushi Bake, 94
rice cakes
    Almond Butter and Banana Rice Cakes, 102
    Cottage Cheese and Avocado Rice Cakes, 102
    Hummus, Turkey, and Cheese Rice Cakes, 102

S

salmon
    Mini Salmon Broccoli Quiche, 138
    Salmon and Cream Cheese Crepes, 136
    Salmon and Cream Cheese Sushi, 128
    Salmon and Cucumber Canapés, 57
    Salmon Sushi Bake, 94
    Teriyaki Salmon and Bok Choy, 44
    Zesty Salmon Power Bowl, 33
seaweed: Salmon Sushi Bake, 94
shallots: Savory Oatmeal with a Poached Egg, 80

shrimp
Crispy Shrimp Rice Paper Rolls, 85
Grilled Shrimp and Zucchini Salad, 54
Red Thai Curry with Shrimp, 92
Shrimp-Stuffed Avocado, 132
spinach
Baked Spinach and Feta Tortilla, 140
Creamy Tuscan Chicken, 49
Egg and Feta Muffins, 129
Green Goddess Smoothie, 112
Italian Meatballs, 47
Mexican-Style Egg Frittata, 32
Mushroom Pearl Couscous, 108
squash: Spaghetti Squash Pizza Nests, 154
sriracha: Salmon Sushi Bake, 94
strawberries
Crepes with Berries and Cream, 158
Greek Yogurt and Berries, 58
Strawberry Oatmeal Smoothie, 114
sunflower seeds
Baklava Bites, 160
Grain-Free Granola, 130
Red Cabbage Slaw, 64
sweet potatoes
One Pan Moroccan Potato Hash, 97
Protein Brownies, 117
Sweet Potato and Turkey Quinoa Bowl, 81
Sweet Potato Avocado Boats, 101
Sweet Potato Fries, 109

T

tahini
Cauliflower Falafel and Tahini Dip, 150–151
Strawberry Oatmeal Smoothie, 114
Veggie Buddha Bowl, 142–143
tea: Sweet 'n Salty Fat Tea Latte, 165
tomatoes
Baked Spinach and Feta Tortilla, 140
Beef and Rice Stuffed Peppers, 98
BLT Pasta Salad, 86
Butter Chicken with Cauliflower Rice, 145
Chicken and Avocado Lettuce Wraps, 42
Chicken Enchiladas, 90–91
Chicken Shish Taouk Skewers, 50
Chili Con Carne, 95
Chop-Chop Salad, 63
Cottage Cheese and Avocado Bowl, 153
Creamy Tuscan Chicken, 49
Egg and Feta Muffins, 129
Fuel-Up Breakfast Burger, 36
Full English Breakfast Quesadilla, 34
Grilled Shrimp and Zucchini Salad, 54
Italian Meatballs, 47
Mexican-Style Egg Frittata, 32
Pesto and Mozzarella Stuffed Chicken, 149
Protein Bento Box, 59
Shakshuka (Eggs Poached in Tomato Sauce), 82
Spaghetti Squash Pizza Nests, 154

Stuffed Cabbage Rolls, 52
Sweet and Sour Beef, 147
Sweet Potato and Turkey Quinoa Bowl, 81
Taco Nachos with Salsa, 88–89
Turkey Stuffed Peppers, 146
Veggie Buddha Bowl, 142–143
Warm Steak Salad, 40
Zesty Salmon Power Bowl, 33
Zucchini and Prosciutto "No Pasta" Lasagna, 148
tortillas
Baked Spinach and Feta Tortilla, 140
Chicken Enchiladas, 90–91
Full English Breakfast Quesadilla, 34
New York Deli Breakfast Burrito, 76
Taco Nachos with Salsa, 88–89
tuna
Tuna and Mayo Topped Baked Potato, 87
Tuna Casserole, 53
turkey
Hummus, Turkey, and Cheese Rice Cakes, 102
Protein Bento Box, 59
Sweet Potato and Turkey Quinoa Bowl, 81
Turkey Stuffed Peppers, 146
turkey bacon
BLT Pasta Salad, 86
Egg Salad Wrap, 43
Full English Breakfast Quesadilla, 34

W

walnuts
Apricot Breakfast Bake, 72
Greek Yogurt and Berries, 58
Stuffed Mushrooms, 69
water chestnuts: Pork San Choi Bao, 39

Y

yogurt
Butter Chicken with Cauliflower Rice, 145
Chicken Shish Taouk Skewers, 50
Frozen Yogurt Bites, 123
Grain-Free Granola, 130
Greek Yogurt and Berries, 58
Green Goddess Smoothie, 112

Z

zucchini
Blueberry and Zucchini Muffins, 60
Grilled Shrimp and Zucchini Salad, 54
Italian Meatballs, 47
Veggie Buddha Bowl, 142–143
Zucchini and Prosciutto "No Pasta" Lasagna, 148
Zucchini Fritters with Fried Eggs, 137